Get back to a happier, healthier you…

ᵀᴴᴱLife Preserver Diet®

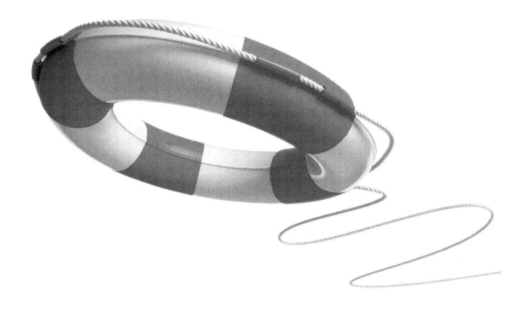

ᴮʸMarcia Berlin, R.D., L.D.
ᵂᴵᵀᴴDeborah Geering

For Quinn, Jim and David.

Contents

Forward

A New Kind of Pampering

I'm sitting outside a coffee shop on a sunny spring day with my co-author, Deborah, as we put the finishing touches on our new book, and we were just saying ... boy, do we feel great! Not just because we are nearing the satisfying conclusion to our two-year journey of writing a book together. But also because we just feel great. Our bodies are well-nourished but not weighing us down. Our hearts and muscles are fit and functioning well — though no one's ever accused us of being fitness freaks. And as we've shaped the messages we wanted to share in this book, we have realized that we are comfortable in our bodies and happy in our outlooks on life (most of the time!).

Don't get the wrong idea. We don't think we're all that and a bag of chips. And we are not super-disciplined rabbit-food eaters who never let ice cream touch our lips, heaven forbid. We're just happy, and pretty healthy, too. It's the result of what we've learned through our experiences: That treating our bodies well is just that — a treat. That healthy foods, healthy living and a do-it-for-myself attitude feel like luxury. That moderate amounts of exercise and a little home cooking ARE possible for busy women, and sometimes even pleasurable.

How do we do it? It's not a trick. It's a mind-set.

What is pampering?

What do you think about when you think of luxury? For me, it's putting my toes in the sand on a little island that I love. With the sun on my shoulders and island music in the air, I am at my happiest. It makes me feel pampered.

We can pamper ourselves in lots of ways, little and big. World cruise? Yup, that counts. So does an afternoon at the hair salon. Or sitting at a café with a friend. Or just watching your teenager finally listen to your instructions and vacuum the living room.

The point is, pampering is doing something that's just for you. This book is about pampering. That's because giving yourself permission to take good care of yourself is a form of pampering.

- It's treating yourself to high-quality, fresh, flavorful foods.

- It's spoiling yourself with organics whenever possible.

- It's setting aside the time to reward your body with what it craves — movement.

- It's learning a few tricks in the kitchen so you can eat food prepared by your favorite chef (you!) instead of relying on junky fast food.

- It's making room for all your favorite treats — including chocolate, or Twinkies, or vegging out in front of the TV — as part of a rewarding lifestyle.

- It's remembering that good food, the pleasure of movement, and a happy attitude should never feel like punishment. They're a luxury that you deserve!

But rarely does a box of pampering just show up on your doorstep. Remember me on the beach with the sand in my toes? I had to get myself there.

Maybe you're not feeling like you're relaxing on a beach right now. Maybe you feel like you're out there with the sharks, drowning in the responsibilities of your life. Who has time for all this pampering?

You do. Really.

Don't worry; I've got a life preserver right here, and I'm tossing it your way and pulling you to shore. (The cabana boy's here with me, and he's got a coconut-shell drink with a little umbrella in it just for you!)

You're gonna get to this happy, healthy place, too. With me and the cabana boy.

But enough about me! Let's talk about you.

Why You? Why Me? Why This Book?

Why you?
Would you describe yourself as being in a sand-in-your-toes kind of place or more like a drowning-with-the-sharks kind of place? My guess, because you are reading this book, is that you can sense the fins circling closer.

Let me take a stab at describing how you have been feeling.

You are tired. You work hard, and you've got a whole lot more to do today before you can crawl into bed and turn out the light. Your kids need you; your husband needs you; possibly your parents need you; maybe you've got a work-related deadline hanging over you, too. You get up every morning and you do everything you can, all day, until you are so tired you can't do any more. And yet, you still feel like you're not doing enough. The PTA wants you to volunteer. Your boss wants you to work later. The house never looks tidy enough. You know you should be cooking dinner more often. Your clothes don't fit.

To top it off, there's that gal down the street. You know who I'm talking about. She always looks totally put-together; her kids never miss the school bus. And where does she find the time to get her nails done? What's wrong with you that you can't keep it together as well as she (apparently) can?

Don't worry about her. She's a freak. She's probably not even real; who knows what's going on behind the scenes there? The truth is, NONE of us has enough time in the day. We're all struggling to meet all of our obligations. And we never, ever feel like we have any time left for ourselves.

If you are reading this book, you are struggling with your weight. You feel as though your overweight comes from a lack of willpower. You are disappointed with yourself for not looking better or feeling better. You've probably tried a million different diets, and even when you did have some success, the weight just popped back on again before you even noticed. You are tired of dieting; tired of feeling fat. You're tired of suggestions from doctors and loved ones that you just need to try a little harder. What you really need, right now, is chocolate.

Am I right? Did I get close? OK, let's talk about me again.

Why me?

I have to tell you a story. It starts with my mother. A Cuban Jew who raised her children in the Chicago suburbs, she was a warm, caring, wise woman with simple tastes and a calming presence. She died at age 42 of breast cancer. When I turned 42, I decided to get tested — for BRCA, the gene mutation whose presence indicates a predisposition for breast cancer. My doctor, Elizabeth Steinhaus, had been after me for a couple years to take the test, but I wasn't sure I wanted to know the answer. If I found out that I tested positive — that I had a genetically high risk to develop breast cancer — what would I do? The only options are to get a double mastectomy or do nothing and see what happens.

Finally, Dr. Steinhaus convinced me, and I took the test. It was positive. The genetic counselor told me I had a 90 percent chance of developing an aggressive form of breast cancer at a young age. I also had a high risk for ovarian cancer.

But by then, I knew exactly what I was going to do. I didn't want to die a young mother in the prime of my life, as my mother did. So I had them take out everything and anything that could kill me. I had a double mastectomy, a hysterectomy, an oopherectomy. But it wasn't ALL fun and games — not everyone thought I should do this. Even though my husband, Jim, was totally supportive, most of my friends thought I was completely out of my mind. They thought I should just monitor to see whether any tumors developed.

But I wanted it all gone. So I underwent surgery in the summer of 2005.

The day I came home from the hospital, Dr. Steinhaus called me. They had biopsied my tissues, and whaddayaknow, they found a tumor. A very small tumor in my right breast, a tumor that had snuck by the mammogram readers — a very aggressive kind, too. If it had been allowed to grow for just six more months, I would have been fighting for my life. Instead, after a few more tests to confirm that the cancer hadn't spread yet, I was scot-free — no chemo, no radiation, no nothing.

It turned out that this was my life-preserver moment. But before I tell you about that, let me go back a little further.

I started out as a professional dancer. You'd think that athletes that use their bodies for a living would take good care of the equipment, but that's not necessarily the case. I lived in a world where people abused their bodies. For instance, in order to look as skinny as possible, they would try to go as long as possible without eating. Or they'd intentionally dehydrate themselves in order to show more muscle definition during a performance.

But like me, they really didn't know what they were doing to their bodies. I used to live on M&Ms and wine. Once, when I had injured my foot, a health food store employee told me to eat nothing but pineapples until it healed. I did it, because he seemed to know what he was talking about.

We dancers did terrible things to our bodies food-wise because we didn't know any better. But somewhere along the way, I decided I wanted facts. Would eating nothing but pineapple really fix my sore foot? I wanted more than hearsay. So I decided to go back to school. I got a degree in nutrition and became a registered dietitian.

As a nutrition counselor, I would see a side of people that they didn't usually show. First of all, they had made the appointment, so they had already decided they wanted help. But then they came into my office, we closed the door, we started to talk … and they poured their hearts out. What I discovered is that lots of overweight people are just like too-skinny dancers! They are unhappy with their bodies, overwhelmed with their lives, and they'll try just about anything to "fix" themselves. Anything, as long is it's quick.

But there's rarely a quick solution to a long-standing problem, now, is there? However, there are sudden insights: life-preserver moments.

Sometimes, when people would come to me with a weight problem, and we would talk about their lives and their responsibilities and their worries — the things that were REALLY driving their unhealthy eating habits — I could actually SEE their life-preserver moment. That's when they suddenly realized that they had been allowing themselves to drown in their day-to-day lives and that getting back to a happier place was within their own control. If you were drowning at sea and someone tossed you a life preserver, you'd probably see that as a pretty big moment. You'd have been given a chance to save yourself, and now all you have to do is act on it. Back in my office, when I'd see people reach their life-preserver moment, I'd give them the facts and motivation they'd need to make healthier choices, and they would make the changes to save themselves.

So, that was my life — helping people identify their unhappy, unhealthy habits; watching them have their life-preserver moments when they took control; and offering nutrition advice so they could become happier and healthier. Then my doctor persuaded me to get that BRCA test done. And I decided, despite many friends' protestations, to have all that surgery. But had I done the right thing? Then I got that post-surgery phone call from my doctor and learned that I had, indeed, had cancer. To be honest, at the time I was too frightened (and angry!) to see it, but later I realized: Choosing surgery had been my life-preserver moment! I had taken control, made a difficult decision, and it had saved my life. I had acted as my own life preserver.

Why this book?

Bookstores are bulging with diet plans. We buy one, read half of it, take the parts we like and follow those guidelines for a while. We learn that dark chocolate contains antioxidants, nuts supply omega-3 fatty acids and fruit has too many carbohydrates. So we stop eating fresh fruit and replace it with chocolate-covered peanuts. When the success doesn't come, we go back to our old habits, with a vengeance. Then we buy another book.

Each year, about 45 million people in the United States go on a diet.[1] The PBS television program "Frontline" reported not too long ago that those dieters spend $40 billion a year on diet books, products and programs.[2] And yet, nearly 130 million adults in the United States are overweight. Almost half of them are considered obese, according to the American Obesity Association.

Does the world really need another diet book? The obesity epidemic is getting worse. In 1991, 12 percent of U.S. adults were considered obese (scoring a 30 or higher on a standard body mass index). By 2001 that figure had grown to 21 percent, according to the National Health Policy Forum. The Febuary 2011 Gallup-Healthways Well-Being Index shows that more than 26 percent of Americans are considered obese — and that more than 63 percent of Americans are considered either obese or overweight.[3]

Fat, obese, chubby, chunky, overweight, whatever word you want to use; too many of us are there.

So yes, the world does need another "diet" book. But it needs one that is actually useful, with practical advice for maintaining a healthy body over a lifetime. One that is scientifically grounded, yet engaging and entertaining. One that really helps us lighten up.

Guess what? Here's that book.

The Life Preserver Diet® offers both helpful advice and a practical tool. The book addresses the daily challenges — and habits and attitudes — that are keeping you out there with the sharks. And it includes a handy tool called the PFD (more on that later) that serves as your life preserver, to help you get back on shore with the sand between your toes. You will feel better, look better and love your life even more.

In the coming chapters, we're going to talk about the things in your life that wear you down and make it hard for you to keep treading water — the things you can't really control. Then we're going to look at the things that ARE in your control — the habits, assumptions and attitudes that are holding you back and keeping you from being your happiest. Next, I'm going to explain the PFD — the little online tool that you use with this book —

and how it will help you make healthier choices about the food you eat. Finally, we'll take some time to talk about the challenges ahead, tips to keep you afloat, and what to do when the waters get choppy.

Now, let's get started.

Worksheet: Your Life-Preserver Moment

Have you had a life-preserver moment? What happened to make you want to take control?

_____

_____

_____

_____

_____

_____

_____

_____

_____

_____

_____

_____

_____

Chapter 1

How Did I Get Here?
Those little lies we tell ourselves

You've decided to get going. You are so ready to get that weight off. How do you begin? The first step is to clear your mind of the kind of thinking that has gotten you where you are today. Delete old messages taking up all that space in your inbox and make room for new ones. Think of this time in your life as the time you start taking control. So stop telling yourself little lies.

No more excuses, no more lies

If you're ready to let go of the unhappy, overweight you, then you must also let go of your old excuses and rationalizations. Excuses may be factual, but they're not helpful. And rationalizations, well, that's just another way of saying that you're lying to yourself.

When it comes to excuses, stop using them! Focus on the things that you can change, not what you can't. You can't change your genes, or the fact that you're going through menopause or that you have thyroid disease. Those are challenges that make losing weight more difficult, but they don't make it impossible. Thinking that the skinny woman in the office is so lucky because she can eat everything she wants is not only a waste of time, but it's also not true. (More on skinny people later — and how they can actually help us!)

We spend so much time talking about the problems that we can talk ourselves out of believing in the solution. If you're really ready to start focusing on the things you can change, then the lies stop here. Being dishonest with ourselves is a major barrier between us and weight loss. When you break down the barrier you will be so much closer! I've heard all sorts of weight-loss lies. Many have come out of my own mouth, in fact. Let me introduce you to a few.

"There's nothing I can do about it."

Many people will go to great lengths to support their denial. For a while, I had a client who is a physician. He is an extremely bright man, a graduate of Harvard Medical School. He came into my office at the hospital wellness center with a stack of papers. They were studies and documents on obesity. All of these studies looked at a connection between obesity and genes. Every week he would spend his hour session with me discussing the possibility that the cause of his weight gain was genetically linked. He spent hours finding research papers to send me. It seemed to me that he could have better spent that time going on walks in his neighborhood instead of working tirelessly to justify being overweight.

I am the first to admit that losing weight takes effort. But sometimes we put more effort into our denial than into trying to fix the problem.

"I only eat grilled chicken, steamed broccoli and brown rice."

This is standard dinner fare for overweight people, apparently. I first learned of this when I was a home health dietitian. I made house calls to people with diabetes, heart disease and obesity. I learned then about diet liars. "I eat 1/2 grapefruit for breakfast, a salad for lunch, no dressing, 3 ounces of grilled chicken, steamed broccoli and a half-cup of brown rice for supper." They're telling me this while I'm sitting at their kitchen table looking at king-size Cheetos and potato chip bags in the trash, Coke cans piled in the garage and Little Debbies in the pantry.

I realized that we all lie to some degree. Mostly to ourselves. Denial just perpetuates the problem. We can't change what we don't know or admit to.

"I exercise all the time."

Exercising and going to the gym are not the same thing. Tell me if this person sounds familiar: She comes into the gym decked out in her finest workout gear — $125 dollar Nike cross trainers, Juicy Couture velour sweat suit, and a towel wrapped around her neck. She's carrying a Starbucks grande café latte and a *People* magazine. She sets the treadmill at low speed and starts walking in slow motion as she sets up her workout station. She's getting her things all situated: her magazine perched on the reading rack and latte in the drink holder. She pauses the treadmill to walk over and say hello to the personal trainers at the fitness desk. (She's never had a session with one, but she's been meaning to.) Ten minutes later, she gets back to her treadmill and sets it on low. She strolls along, fixes her hair, flips through the magazine and sips her coffee for about 10 more minutes. She picks up her phone and sends a few text messages. Then, her phone rings and she talks for five minutes, still slow-motion walking. She looks at her watch and says to the person on the phone, "Oh, look at the time. I've been here 45 minutes, I gotta go — I'll see ya tonight at the Cheesecake Factory." She hangs up the phone, gathers her things and runs out of the gym at lightning speed. (The most strenuous part of her workout.)

Do any of these lies sound familiar? Ever heard them? Ever said them? It's OK; you're among friends here. We've all been there.

Time to face the fat

So you've gotten a little, or a lot, overweight. Don't beat yourself up about it. It happened. It's OK ... let's face the fat. Now, together. Denial is a common problem among people who have trouble reversing unhealthy habits. (According to researchers from the University of Texas Southwestern Medical Center, a substantial proportion of obese people didn't think that they needed to lose weight.[4]) If we are not ready or willing to face facts, we bury our heads in the sand. We figure if we can't see it, maybe it's not real and we don't have to deal with it.

Sometimes I get in the shower when I only have 10 minutes to get out of the house. Now realistically, there's no way that I can accomplish this. But once I'm in the shower, I can't see a clock — so, time has stopped, right? I enjoy my long, luxurious shower. But when I get out, I panic when I actually look at a clock and I know how late I am.

Same goes if we never get on a scale. If we can't see how much we weigh, we don't really have to think about being overweight. Or if we camouflage our weight with oversized clothes, we don't have to see the weight we've gained. We even take it a step further — once we do see how much we weigh, we come up with excuse after excuse. But inevitably, the truth comes out. Sometimes, it comes from an undeniable statement from a physician or loved one. Sometimes, it comes right from us.

My moment of truth came one Thanksgiving eve. I'm standing

in front of the mirror about to brush my teeth. Usually for bed I wear an extra large, comfy T-shirt. But tonight, I put on my special, holiday-best pajamas. "It's all about you" is what they say on the shirt and all over the pants. We're visiting relatives, which is why I had to put on my best jammies.

Whoa, what happened here? My cutest jammies don't look so darling anymore. They look like they belong to ... someone much smaller than me. I'm pouring out of them; they look like sausage casing. I somehow have become one big sausage. They must've shrunk. And this is probably a fat mirror.

I go to the guest bedroom, with a normal mirror. Hmm ... still looks the same, that's weird, that my relatives would have two fat mirrors in their house. Back in the bathroom, I start brushing my teeth, and it hits me ... wait a minute; could I have grown? But how? I'm a professional dancer! Well OK, so that was 10 years ago. But I'm an avid exerciser. I go to the gym regularly — well, I did until my membership ran out about a year ago.

I sit on the bed and start thinking about what could have gone wrong. Last week I did buy the same pants that I bought last year, but one size bigger. I told myself that I now like bigger clothes in the winter, and I actually believed me at the time. I remember standing on my scale a couple weeks ago and it was 10 pounds more than last time I weighed myself, maybe six months before that. I convinced myself at the time that the scale was old. I didn't accuse it of being old and out of whack when I liked what I weighed.

Now all the things I've been putting out of my mind come flooding back. My clothes used to complement my curves, my small waist. Now what's with my clothes? They're moving my bottom to just above my hips (a place that should have no name because it's not supposed to be there), and just-above-my-hips are overflowing out of my low-rise jeans. That's a nice look.

Am I overweight? It hits me … hard. I'm a fatty! It's Thanksgiving eve and I'm a fatty, in pajamas that don't fit me anymore. And I'm supposed to stuff myself tomorrow. I run for my calendar and start flipping through pages. Next week is my office holiday party; a week later, I'm going to a Hanukkah party. A week after that are three Christmas parties, then New Year's Eve, Chinese New Year …. I keep flipping: Valentine's Day, my husbands birthday, Easter, Passover (I am in a multicultural family), my birthday, end of the school year luau, family reunion, Fourth of July … It's not looking good. Oh wait, look at August — I got nothing in August. That'll be the time to start eating right and exercising. I'm going to make some serious changes in August! It will be perfect, less temptations, I'll start then.

Just then my daughter, who was then seven, walks in and asks what I'm looking for in the calendar. "Oh, just a time when there's no special occasions or holidays so I can start my new eating and exercise plan," I say.

"Mom, there's always special occasions and holidays. Why don't you start now? Duh." And she walks out of the room. Shouldn't she be in bed?

It's true, there are always special occasions and holidays. Every day is Thanksgiving. Granted, we don't always have feasts, but we do always have something going on to tempt us. So I decide to revise my August start date. It's time to start now. I'll see if I can get through Thanksgiving without busting my casing. Then I'll make a plan on Friday.

A new day, a new way

Facing the fat can be scary. It's scary because once we face the reality, then we know it's time to take action. Once we take action, we start remembering past failures. This time, failure is not an option. Trust me, this time will be different — it will stick. You've got a life preserver. You will start giving yourself the TLC you need to get your body where it should be. You'll be pampering yourself with delicious, wholesome food and energizing, refreshing exercise.

Your way of doing things will become the old way. It won't be part of your reality anymore. Gone are the days where you dread dieting because it means sacrificing and suffering. In the chapters ahead you will learn to enjoy the process.

So right now, say it loud, and say it proud. Don't let excuses and lies and denial stop you. "I'm fat! I'm mad as hell and I'm not gonna take it anymore!"

That's right, sister. So let's see what your new life is going to look like.

Worksheet: The Moment of Truth

Overweight doesn't happen overnight. How did you get here? Tell the truth — I won't judge!

_____

_____

_____

_____

_____

The truth feels good, doesn't it! What little lies have you been telling yourself about your eating and exercise habits?

_____

_____

_____

_____

_____

Now they they're out there, they lose their power. They won't hold you back any longer.

Chapter 2

What Skinny People Do

I was sitting in the office of my favorite doctor, Dr. Steinhaus. I like her because she saved my life. She's the surgeon who talked me into having the breast cancer gene test. This was the first appointment I had had with her since my reconstruction. I was excited to show her the new me. When she walked in, I saw a new her — she had lost a bunch of weight. She looked great.

After we hugged and I thanked her for the whole life-saving thing, I asked her how she had lost the weight and become so strong, fit, healthy and lean. "I do what skinny people do," she told me. She explained that she had started watching skinny people and copying them. Dr. Steinhaus got me thinking. I started watching them, too. Theirs are the footsteps we want to follow.

A few weeks later, my daughter and I went to Chicago to visit family and friends. The first stop was the penthouse. My brother Gerry and his wife Francina have this great penthouse condo in the South Loop. You can see their living room window from Lake Shore Drive. Francina is incredibly fit for a 40-something accountant. She always looks great in her Anne Taylor suits. She's so fit, she looks like a teenager. I thought of Dr. Steinhaus and her plan to watch skinny people. Francina qualifies, so I watched.

Francina and Gerry have an ultra-cool urban lifestyle. Every day, we ate at fabulous restaurants within walking distance of their place. I noticed that Francina had an unusual ordering system.

"I'll have the vegetable croissant sandwich and a side of turkey sausage," she told the waitress at a little breakfast place we went to. She left half of the croissant on her plate and ate half of an order of sausage. My niece ate the rest of the sausage. She didn't bring home the sandwich because she's doesn't really care for leftovers.

At dinner, Francina and Gerry split an entrée, and Gerry ordered an appetizer for himself.

Francina custom orders. She gets creative with restaurant ordering to help maintain her weight. She's not shy about it, and she does it every time she eats out. If the menu doesn't meet her needs, she makes some changes and *voila* … custom ordering. Francina allows herself to eat out regularly but has a habit of eating all of her food in moderation.

One night, we all walked to Grant Park to watch a movie. We were sitting in the grass, and I noticed that Francina was wearing some cute jeans. "I love those!" I told her and touched the bottoms of her jeans. I felt something on her ankles. "What is that? I asked. And she showed me — ankle weights. She wore them on our walk to the park. We weren't going on a power walk or anything. She told me that she wears them on most days to keep her leg muscles strong. She wears them around the house, to the office, just anywhere.

Hmm. So this is what skinny people are up to! So far, I've got **Skinny people custom order at restaurants,** and **Skinny people take advantage of even tiny opportunities to exercise.** Who would've thought to wear ankle weights even when you're not at the gym? I love it. What a great way to fit exercise into your everyday life.

On the same trip, my daughter and I traveled to the suburbs to stay with a friend of the family, Gloria. She has a beautiful old house, one of those 100-year-old grand dames on a wooded lot. She was a very gracious host and happens to be a skinny person, too. The day we arrived, Gloria ran out to the grocery store. When she came back, she had bags and bags of food.

"I didn't know if you guys liked green or red grapes, so I got both," she said as she was unloading the bags. "And doesn't this watermelon look beautiful?" The fridge was stocked with fresh fruit, lunch meat, salad fixings and yogurt. The pantry was filled with all different kinds of high-fiber cereal, nuts, multigrain bread and gourmet chocolate. I told Gloria that she didn't have to do that for us. She said, "Oh, my kitchen is always well-stocked. I like to have a little bit of everything for me and whoever might stop by."

Her kitchen was not only well-stocked but it was also such a happy place to be. It was one of those kitchens that's lived in, full of activity and where everyone ends up hanging out. Now I've got something else to add to the list. **Skinny people keep a kitchen well-stocked with healthy foods.** To Gloria, food is something to be celebrated and enjoyed. There are always healthy food choices available — and some treats, carefully chosen. She eats nourishing, satisfying food on a regular basis. And she occasionally indulges in something more extravagant that she really loves, like fancy chocolate. It keeps her in the habit of balanced eating.

Back in Georgia, I was still doing my research on what skinny people do. I went to my friend Wendy's house one Sunday afternoon. Wendy is a 30-something woman with a family of four to feed. I was just in time to catch her doing her weekly menu plan. On her kitchen table she had her calendar, recipes, paper and pen. She checked the calendar, saw what activities were going on on certain days of the week and planned accordingly. Then we went off to the grocery store with our list for all of the meals. She puts the week's meal plan on the fridge so her family can get dinner started if she'll be coming home late on a given night.

More skinny-people tricks: **They plan meals ahead.** Wendy tells me that her mother had always done the same thing, and without a plan she'd be lost. This way, all of the decisions are made before the week even starts. She incorporates a variety of foods and includes her family in meal preparation.

I was in my backyard recently, talking to my neighbor Grace. Judging by her trim, fit figure, you'd never know she gave birth to three children. Our kids were jumping on the trampoline and showing us their tricks. Her husband, Al, pulled up in their driveway with groceries. He was unloading the bags and Grace said, "Make sure you leave the powdered donuts in the car." I thought that was interesting. "Is he bringing them somewhere?" I asked. "Oh no, I just have no control when it comes to powdered donuts — so they stay in the car, for him," she answered.

Good Grace-ism, I thought. And another skinny-person trick: **They avoid irresistible junk foods.** I started asking more questions. Is there anything else he leaves in the car? "Girl Scout cookies. But those go to his office ... they'll melt in the car. But chocolate brownies that come in a box, I don't like that fake chocolate, so those can come in the house," she said.

I told Grace I needed to do more research on her, so she invited us to stay for dinner. Research does have its perks.

I watched her prepare plates for Al, the kids and herself. Her husband's plate had more food on it than hers. "I know that I can't eat like a man, so I make sure to give myself more appropriate portions," she explained. When dining out or eating at someone else's house, women and men do usually get served the same portions. At restaurants, I guess, it might cause a riot if the server brought smaller meals for women than men, but that really would make more sense. In general, men are able to consume more calories and still maintain their body weight. So when eating at home, women should make it a point to not eat like a typical man.

I asked Grace to tell me more about her eating habits. She told me that she used to cook one meal for her husband and kids and prepare something different for herself. For example, she would make fried chicken for him and the kids, while she ate baked chicken. But she realized that it would be healthier for the whole family to eat baked chicken, so now that's what they all have. On occasion, she'll fry or make "oven-fried" chicken as a compromise.

That night at dinner, Grace was the last one to sit down to eat because she was the chef and server. She was also the last one to finish. "I take my time so I can tell when I'm satisfied," she said. "If I try to hurry up and finish when everyone else does, I overstuff myself — and I hate that feeling," she told me. **Skinny people serve themselves appropriate portions, and they savor their meals.**

After dinner, I helped her clean up. Then she said, "Now I usually go for a walk." "Don't you need to put the kids to bed?" I asked.

She told me that she and Al have a system in which she cooks and cleans the kitchen, and he gets the kids ready for bed. "I take care of everybody else all day long," she said. "Going for a walk at the end of the day is something I do just for me." We went for a walk in the neighborhood. I hadn't done anything for myself that day either. It felt good.

I can't forget to mention Barb. I don't know who came first, Barb or Martha Stewart. Barb always has beautifully arranged fresh flowers in each room of her house. She's got delightfully scented soaps in the bathrooms, uses cloth napkins for every meal and has environmentally friendly, high-thread-count sheets on her beds. She throws great parties, is a successful businesswoman, volunteers for several nonprofit organizations, is a wife and mother and a dear friend of mine, and she's — you guessed it — in great shape. And she's actually nice!

One unique habit of Barb's is that she collects workout DVDs. There is not another collection out there that can match it. She's got cardio kick boxing, belly dancing, yogalates, step aerobics, Latin dance party … any workout DVD that's ever come out, she's got it. And the great thing is that she actually uses them. She religiously does a 30-minute workout DVD every weekday morning. She's a busy woman and likes the convenience, the variety and the alone time. Since she uses them repeatedly, she gets really good at them. It's always more fun to do something you're good at. **Barb, a skinny person, found an exercise plan that fits her lifestyle.**

And here's one for the men: my friend Ed. He weighs the same now as when I met him 20 years ago. He's always been athletic. Played sports as a kid and through college. He still exercises but much less than he did when he was younger. Most of us 40-somethings do less exercise than we used to. He rehabs homes for a living. So, he's active and has a physical job. I asked Ed what keeps him so lean and mean. "I don't pig out anymore," he said. "Those days are gone."

"That's it?" I asked.

"That's it." **Skinny people like Ed adapt their eating habits as their bodies age.**

What do all these people have in common? Are they perfect? No, of course not. Do they ever get off track? Absolutely; they are human. Do they all have the same lifestyle? No, they're all extremely different. But, there is one skinny thread that ties them all together. They are in charge. They take care of themselves in a way that works for them.

10 skinny-people tips

1. Custom order at restaurants. Remember the movie "When Harry Met Sally?" Sally was a custom-ordering queen; Francina is too. She makes up her own menu. She calls the shots when eating out. She knows that restaurant portions are too big. So she not only leaves some of the food on her plate, but she also mixes and matches menu items so that she gets what she really wants. Don't be afraid to be different. Go against the grain a little.

2. Fit exercise in where you can, and choose a plan that fits your lifestyle. It takes a little creativity, like wearing ankle weights or negotiating with your spouse for a "me-time" walk in the evening. The gym is not the only place to get a workout. Run up and down the stairs a few times a day; put some hand weights in your office and do a set while you're talking on the speaker phone. Whatever works for you.

Barb the domestic diva takes it upon herself to squeeze exercise into her hectic schedule. She knows how limited her time is, and she doesn't even entertain the thought of taking more than 30 minutes out of her day to exercise. She's created an environment where she can go to her personal DVD workout library, choose what she wants, and she's through in half an hour.

3. Keep a well-stocked, healthy kitchen. When you have plenty of delicious, healthy food in your house, you don't need to go out for every meal. Let food bring joy into your home, like Gloria does with her happy kitchen. She fills her kitchen with foods that she enjoys and that are good for her.

Often times I hear clients say to me, "I just eat whatever's in the fridge," and I say, "Whatever's in the fridge? Who puts it there?" Take charge and fill your refrigerator with foods that you really want. Don't just fill it with diet foods because commercials tell you to. Or, even worse, don't let your pantry go bare, leaving you at the mercy of fast-food restaurants.

4. Plan meals. It sounds easy enough. But it must be easier said than done, or we'd all do it. Weekly plans are a good idea, but if you have to do it twice a week to start … that's OK, too. Baby steps.

Prioritize and make time for what's most important to you. Wendy, the master planner, knows that it is a priority for her to enjoy a nice family dinner every night. So she makes it happen.

Her Sunday planning session is how she ensures there will be spaghetti and Caesar salad on Wednesday night.

5. Keep no-can-do foods out of the house. You know those snacks that you just can't have a little of? Keep them out of reach — unless you happen to be crazy for celery. Understand what works or doesn't work for you. Grace, the supermom, takes action by sending her trigger foods out to the car with her husband.

6. Choose treats for your kids that you don't care for. That way, the kids aren't deprived of treats and you aren't tempted. Many of us are guilty of blaming the children for the presence of certain foods in the house: "I need to have chocolate chip cookies in the house for my kids." Your kids probably like sour gummy worms just as much, even if you don't.

7. Only eat like a man if you are one. Men typically need 400 to 500 more calories per day than women. For that reason alone, in my next life I hope to come back as a man. But this rule applies to body size as well as gender — so coming back as a really tall woman would work, too! If you have a small frame, male or female, you're going to need fewer calories than a person with a large frame. Sorry, but them's the breaks. Try to console yourself with the knowledge that in a famine, big people go hungry sooner.

8. Eat slowly. It just makes sense that if you wolf down your food, it will be gone before you have had a chance to enjoy it. But there's a scientific reason why savoring your food is good for you, too. When you eat, your stomach tells your brain that it's full. Your brain then tells you that you're full. But the problem is, it takes about 20 minutes for this response to kick in. So, if you eat too quickly, your food is gone, literally, before you know it — before your body knows it's been fed. To make matters worse, if you are multitasking while you eat, you're not even paying attention to your brain as it tries to tell you, "Stop eating already; you're full and about to overflow."

9. Reward yourself with a healthy break. Do something just for you every day — something like a walk in the evening, a disco-dance study break, or anything else you enjoy. Are we all so important that the world will stop spinning if we have a little fun for a few minutes? If I pull out my Hula Hoop at the office, I'm pretty sure my company will stay in business.

10. Don't pig out anymore. Those days are gone. Ed, the regular guy, isn't sitting back and accepting weight gain just because he's getting older. He's taking charge and facing reality. He just can't eat as much as he used to.

Remember the old saying, "You can never be too rich or too thin"? It's not all true. We aren't looking to be too thin. Strong, fit, healthy and lean is the goal here. Now, I don't know about the "too rich" part. But I may start watching what rich people do next, so that I can follow in their footsteps, too.

Chapter 3

The Outside World

The purpose of this chapter is to help you gain a better understanding of what is working against you in the outside world, pinpoint the everyday pitfalls and give basic survival tips. Then in Chapters 6, 7 and 8, we'll get into more detail about strategies for winning the battle.

In this chapter we will take a look around and see that it's really rough out there. There's so much working against us. It's not entirely your fault. Our obesogenic (creating obesity) society and environment have made it increasingly difficult to stay at a healthy weight. It's almost impossible to resist continuously gaining weight if we don't have a strategy to fight it and the tools to guide us. It's not just you; you're living in a crazy world.

So give yourself a break, grab a cup of tea, and continue reading. Let's talk about the outside world and why we face such a never-ending battle to lose weight.

In order to fight and come out a winner, we must understand the enemy. This is a war on weight, and the enemy is out there, just waiting to attack when we least expect it.

"If you know the enemy and know yourself," China's Sun Tzu advised in the 6th century B.C., "you need not fear the results of a hundred battles."

So let's get to know the enemy.

Enemy No. 1: Big friendly cows

Anything for a buck. Have we no shame? Junk food sells. That is why almost every place we go has junk food for sale. Kids like junk, so schools sell junk.

Friday is Chick-fil-A day at my daughter's school. For a fund-raiser, they sell hot chicken biscuit sandwiches from the fast-food chain in the car pool lane. Every Friday my daughter gets out of the car and pays her $2 for a deep-fried chicken biscuit. The vendor, dressed in a cow suit, smiles and waves to the parents in the cars while the kids buy their biscuits. I give Quinn a kiss, let her out of the car, and give the cow a dirty look as I drive away. As a nutritionist and a mom, I can't stand this Friday tradition or that big, friendly cow. But I tell myself it's only once a week, and I drive off to work.

One Friday, Quinn forgot her library book in the car after I dropped her off. So I parked the car and went in to bring her the book. I'm not usually in school in the morning, so I was enjoying walking through the halls. I saw two little girls pulling a red wagon full of blue and red boxes, stopping at each classroom. When they got closer, I realized that the boxes were Krispy Kreme doughnut boxes. "Oh, is it doughnut day or something?" I asked, wondering why there would be a doughnut day on Chick-fil-A day. "Every day is doughnut day," they told me, and rolled on.

Another fund-raiser. Unbelievable. On my way out of school I noticed on the walls that there was the same poster in every hallway. It was an Otis Spunkmeyer cookie poster with a picture of a darling little girl hugging a giant chocolate chip cookie. Another fund-raiser. Is there no other way we can raise money for our schools? Bombarded with so much junk food, all before 8 a.m. And why? Because it's in the best interest of the children? No — because junk food sells.

Adults are pummeled with similar messages, in similar ways. There may not be a guy in a cow suit at your office, but there's probably someone selling doughnuts — maybe even cubicle to cubicle. And the nearest biscuit-dealer is likely just a few hundred yards away.

Survival tips: We don't have to give in to the cow. I can limit my child to buying a chicken biscuit to twice a month instead of weekly. I can also explain why: "It's not a healthy habit to get into every week." I tell myself the same thing. (And because that cow gets on Mommy's nerves.)

Enemy No. 2: Mun-ching

When I went to China, I saw hundreds of people in the park doing tai chi early in the morning, before the workday began. They would ride their bikes to the park, do tai chi and then ride to work. There was not a fat person in the bunch.

What do we Americans do in the morning? Instead of tai chi-ing, we prefer mun-ching. This is where, instead of riding our bikes to a park, we drive our cars up to a window, pick up a fried sausage sandwich, and then begin munching. In our society, why haven't we carved out time to exercise? We have such sedentary lifestyles that we can go days without moving anything but fingers on computer keyboards. Worksite wellness is starting to surface, but it's not nearly enough. If we don't incorporate exercise into our days, our days will be numbered. Workplace obesity costs $73.1 billion a year, according to a 2010 study published in the *Journal of Occupational & Environmental Medicine.*[5]

Survival tips: Take it upon yourself to fit exercise in. Find walking buddies at the office or neighborhood and walk together at lunch. Talk to your human resources department about a worksite wellness program. Take a break every hour or two from your desk and stretch or move around.

Enemy No. 3: The office candy trap

The candy dish is a thing of the past. The word "dish" brings to mind a small, pretty decoration that sits on a side table in your living room filled with a handful of colorful hard candy. The office candy dish is actually a trap. Every office has at least one. The trap is placed strategically on the desk of the trapper. She sets out a colossal, bottomless pit of the most decadent candy. She will not usually eat any herself. No, the trapper sits back and takes pleasure in watching co-workers being lured in throughout the day. She gets great satisfaction out of refilling her bait again and again. She knows that where there is candy, the people will come.

Why? Maybe she wants to fatten up the people around her so she looks thinner; maybe she wants to live vicariously through others; or maybe she just likes to have people visit her desk. The reason she became a trapper is irrelevant. Just beware, because she is relentless. The candy trap is always waiting to snag you.

Not that I'm against candy. But the trap is a whole different animal. It beckons you at your weakest moments and is disguised as innocent pleasure, but it's deadly. What harm could there be in a few little Hershey's Kisses, you ask? It's the kiss of death if you go back time after time during the day. That can add up to several hundred calories, equivalent to an extra meal that you're eating each day. Don't get trapped.

Survival tips: Keep track of how much you take, or stay away. Don't let it sneak up on you. Bring your own snacks to have on hand.

Enemy No. 4: FedEx syndrome

We must have it now, right now!

When I give a presentation or workshop on nutrition I ask my audience why we're not eating properly. What's keeping us from healthy eating? Without fail the answer is, "No time."

Why do we have no time to eat properly? My theory: It's because of FedEx. We do things super-fast to save time. Since we're saving so much time, we can do more. Now that we're expected to do so much more, we have less time.

With its overnight mail, FedEx is part of a trend. The *I want it now* trend. Everything sped up from there. Technology is faster, mail is instant, but our brains are the same. They don't go any faster. Our brains can't keep up, so we end up spinning out of control. We get overwhelmed because in one day we've sent so many more messages, more projects are due, and more texts need to be answered. We have our Blackberrys or our iPhones with us for every waking moment. There's no time to breathe, and take things in, digest information, mull it over. We can't even say, "The check's in the mail" anymore. Things are expected to be done immediately now. There's no calling in sick, either, because you're expected to use the company laptop or take a conference call while you're at home.

With everything moving so fast, it's no wonder we have no time to prepare and eat a decent meal. We've lost control of our schedules. We have set up ourselves so that we have no choice but to eat whatever's closest and fastest. I like technology as much as anybody, but we can have our technology and eat, too!

Survival tips: Put your foot down. You don't have to work when you're sick or get projects finished in record time. It's not a race. Don't answer your phone all the time. Put down the Crackberry and chill once in a while. Make yourself dinner.

Enemy No. 5: Showroom kitchens

When you walk into a new home these days, they always have fancy kitchens: marble countertops, glass-door cabinets, stainless-steel appliances. They're so beautiful, no one wants to get them dirty. So, often, they just sit there, gleaming and unused, while the family orders take-out.

Eating is an afterthought. Very rarely do families gather at the dinner table, and even more rarely has anyone planned out the meal. Instead, we tend to grab our food on the go or from a microwavable box in the freezer. We've developed unhealthy eating behaviors that reflect our crazy-busy lifestyles: mindless eating, eating on the fly and skipping meals.

- Mindless eating is when you multitask while you eat, preventing you from really noticing and enjoying your food. So you eat more. I also call this the where-is-my-Pop-Tart syndrome. I was eating a chocolate fudge Pop Tart, an indulgence I allow myself occasionally, while I was walking around doing other stuff. A few minutes later, I asked my husband, "Where'd my Pop Tart go?" He said, "Uh, you ate it, Marcia." I looked around, and sure enough, it was gone. Bummer. I didn't enjoy it because I didn't even notice I was eating it. I got robbed — calories with no enjoyment. That is mindless eating. So instead we need to sit down, eat and enjoy.

- Eating on the fly is when we leave meals to chance, impulse eating. We are at the mercy of fast-food chains. Fast-food restaurants make their fortunes off of grab-n-go eaters. There's no time for anything else, so we go to a drive-through. The fast-food restaurants have made it even more convenient by accepting credit cards. Fast-food chains are very savvy when it comes to taking our money.

- Meal-skippers gain weight. First of all, if you're not hungry for breakfast, you've likely eaten too much the night before. We should be hungry in the morning, at least for something small. Second, skipping meals causes you to overeat at your next meal; there's no getting around it. Third, skipping meals puts your body in a starvation mode, which slows your metabolism. If our metabolism is working properly, we should be hungry every few hours.

Survival tips: Admit to yourself that you need to make changes and commit to making them. Plan your meals ahead of time, pack your lunch the night before, sit when you eat, have an eating cut-off time at night. Take control.

Enemy No. 6: The television set

You've got that fabulous 42-inch flat-screen TV that you bought with your tax refund last year. The picture looks great. But does it have to be the center of your universe? In almost every American home the first thing you notice, from just about any angle, is the television set. When a TV is the focal point of someone's home, the message is clear: It's likely to also be the focal point of the family's life.

Take a moment to think about all the dreams and plans you have. Is "watching more TV" one of them? And yet, so many of us come home after a long day of work, switch on the box in the center of our living rooms, and never get back up off the sofa.

Survival tips: Here's a suggestion: One night a week, don't turn the TV on. What will you do with all that time? Read a book? Go on a bike ride? Take a bath? Have a conversation with a family member? Pretty much anything you decide to do will probably make you feel a lot better than will another lost evening in front of the television set.

What? Miss an episode of "Celebrities in Their Underwear"? All I can say to you is, the first step toward recovery is acknowledging you have a problem. If there's no way you can turn off the TV for a whole evening because you just CAN'T miss your show, then you might want to stop and think about that. Will your life really come to a screeching halt if you miss one episode? You'll probably be able to pick up the story line next week. But tonight, treat yourself to something special. When you choose to do things just for you, you feel more in control of your life as a whole — and you realize that you really do have time to take better care of yourself, too.

Enemy No. 7: Aliens

There are these foreign beings surrounding us. They are on billboards, magazines, movies and TV. They are disguised as leggy super models. But I'm here to tell you that they are freaks of nature; they are not normal humans from this planet. They are proportioned completely differently than humans. Why would we compare ourselves to aliens? It's impossible to be them — they are not of our species. Victoria Secret models are stick figures with breasts (and sometimes wings). Their purpose is to make us Earthlings feel bad about ourselves. We need to set more realistic goals and find more realistic role models. Remember, we're trying to do what skinny people do, not what aliens do.

Survival tips: Buy magazines that have a positive impact on your life — cooking, healthy living or travel, for instance. Find positive role models whom you admire. Work out and get muscles so if you run into one of these super models one day, you can challenge her to arm wrestle and show her who's really in control — and what a truly healthy body can do.

Enemy No. 8: Fat is the new normal

According to a study published in the academic journal Economic Inquiry, increased obesity in the population has led to even more weight gain as our perception of what is considered a normal body size has changed.[6]

Have you noticed that a size 12 now isn't what a size 12 used to be? Sizing is much more generous than it was just 10 years ago. That's called "vanity sizing," and clothes manufacturers do it all the time. They know you'd rather be a size 12 than a size 14, so they call the size 14 — or even a 16 — a 12, and scale everything from there. You may be proud of your "new" size, but are you really at a healthy weight for your body?

If people around us are overweight, then we may talk ourselves into thinking that we're not really overweight; we're normal. Fat is the new normal. When we hang out with fat people, we don't feel as fat, relatively speaking. And speaking of relatives …

Getting together with the Jewish/Cuban side of my family was always entertaining. The Jewbans are a colorful group. My grandma cracked everybody up. Like most old ladies, she wasn't afraid to speak her mind. And she did so in her Yiddish, Spanish, broken English accent. So almost anything she said sounded funny — like "happy gabuzday" instead of "happy birthday."

One time I brought a friend of mine with me to a family reunion. I said, "Grandma, this is my friend Beth." She said, "Nice to meet you Beth. I'm fat, you're fat, I like you," and gave her a big hug. We all had a laugh, including Beth, and I didn't think much of it, because it was just like my grandma to blurt out uncensored thoughts. Now, I think I know why she was so happy to meet good-natured Beth. Most of the Jewban side of my family were fit and trim. So my Grandma stuck out because she was overweight. When Beth came along, my grandma wasn't the only one.

Survival tips: Instead of comparing yourself to others, raise the bar and strive to be your personal best.

These are just eight enemies that I've identified. You may have others. Maybe your mother-in-law drives you to eat excessively. Maybe the ice cream store on your block is calling to you. Think about the people, places and things that keep you from meeting your weight-loss goals. They may change or stay the same over time. The important thing is that we all realize it is not easy out there, and you must be streetwise to survive.

Now that we've identified our enemies, what can we do about them? First, know that you can do this. You can lose weight and keep it off. You just have to take it one step at a time. There are no shortcuts. Second, surround yourself with a supportive environment to balance out our obesogenic culture. Not all restaurants have giant portions. There are some where every meal is low-calorie. At a chain of restaurants called Seasons 52, for example, all meals are less than 475 calories. Take advantage of the take-out counters at health-oriented grocery stores. Shop at farmers' markets; it will motivate you to get back to eating food with integrity. Become part of the wellness culture, and you'll see that the world around us does have places that support your goal. They may be in the minority, but they are out there.

Preparation is paramount. You know that there's fast food on every corner; you know most meals you get are super-sized; you know that you're too busy to cook when you get home. So prepare. You bought this book, didn't you? You're reading it, and you're ready to make all the preparations to help you move forward. Don't support fast-food chains anymore. Don't get suckered in to doing things that go against your grain. You are stronger than the enemies. Surround yourself with people, places and things that help you meet your goals. Start using some of these survival tips, and you'll be well on your way to a lifetime of weight management. Nothing can stop you. Not even a big, friendly cow.

Chapter 4

Inside of You

It's 6:45 a.m. My alarm goes off, alarmingly loud. After my shower, I'm standing in my closet wrapped in a towel, brushing my teeth and staring at the clothes hanging in front of me. I drift off, picturing myself when I used to look great in these clothes. I think about how much money I spent on them. I scan from one end of the closet to the other, stopping at each item: too tight, too tight, way too tight. I remember the time I went out dancing with my girlfriends, and those designer jeans were perfect with that low-cut top. There's the linen suit I wore to give that presentation at work.

I let out a long sigh. I have nothing to wear today. I hate my clothes. I hate my body. My fat butt will never get back into these clothes. I hear Matt Lauer's voice; it must be 7:30. I grab my black pants with the elastic waist and a long top, throw a jacket over it. I check myself in the mirror to make sure my body is hidden. Now, I've got no time for breakfast, so I grab a honey bun at the cafeteria when I get to work and hate myself for it. What a way to start the day.

Self-defeating habits

Stuart Smalley, the self-help-addicted character Al Franken used to play before he was a U.S. senator, was onto something with his "stinkin' thinkin'" philosophy. Many of us start off our days a lot like this, feeling hopeless and focusing on the negative.

Talking trash to ourselves. We talk to ourselves negatively, with
no respect. We wouldn't dare talk to anyone else that way. So why
is it OK to do that to ourselves?

When we start the morning this way, where's the inspiration?
We need to feel ready to take on the day in a positive way. We
need confidence that we can meet our goals. Instead we're barely
getting by, happy to just to make it through another one. We're
unsure of our ability to lose weight, so we tend to settle. Doubting
ourselves can lead to failure. "Any ounce of doubt is self-defeat,"
my personal trainer, Roger, likes to say.

Here are some self-defeating habits that keep us from meeting
our goals:

Being too hard on ourselves: If you say things like, "I'm so fat
it's disgusting, and it will never change. I have no will power —
I'm such a loser," then you need to cut yourself a break. You've
quit before you've even begun. Acknowledge that there's room for
improvement, and then start working on it.

Being too easy on ourselves: On the other hand, if you say
things like, "It's not my fault; there's no way I have time to cook
or exercise, and I'm really not that far gone anyway, most people
are about my size," then you are letting yourself off the hook too
easily. As important as it is to recognize the outside forces that are
working against us, it's just as critical to accept responsibility for
our own good health.

Assuming that getting older means getting out of shape: I was
on the elliptical machine at the gym one morning, feeling really
good about my 20 minutes of cardio. Bill, who was 87 years old

at the time, was next to me. He was a regular at the gym since his heart attack. Bill carefully monitored his heart rate as he exercised. I was about to step off the machine when I realized that Bill and I had gotten on at the same time, and he was still going strong. I got back on and kept going until five minutes after Bill got off. I'd be damned if an 87-year-old cardiac rehab patient would outlast me! That's when I realized that I want to be like Bill when I grow up. Getting old is all relative.

Missing the forest for the trees: Program diets are supposed to be shortcuts for healthy eating, not excuses for cheating. Sure, some diets may suggest that pork rinds are "OK." But are they? Is it ever good for your body to fill it with a bag of mostly grease? Pork rinds may be low in carbohydrates, but that does not mean they are anywhere near healthy or nourishing for your body.

What other "trees" have we come to accept while completely missing the "forest" of healthy eating? There are many, many outrageous behaviors we've come to accept as appropriate. One diet "rule" out there is to not eat white foods. White foods are not the enemy; it's when we eat mostly white foods that they become a problem. And what kind of white foods are we talking about? A baked potato, white rice, white pasta, French bread … none of those foods will kill us. They just have to be part of a bigger plan. If we load up our baked potatoes, white rice, white pasta or French bread with veggies and lean protein, the white stuff becomes a part of a balanced meal.

Meanwhile, some of the same people who doggedly dodge white foods eat frozen packaged meals, often loaded with sodium, sugar and other additives, on a daily basis. Whole foods from the earth, even potatoes, are healthy. The boxed foods with ingredients that we can't pronounce; those are the foods we don't want to fill up on. When clients tell me that they're off of white food and instead eat a frozen, processed packaged meal every day, I think they've missed the forest for the trees.

Now, I am not totally knocking frozen meals. There are some that are minimally processed, and they do have a place. I have many clients tell me that they go out for fast food every day for lunch because of the convenience. When I recommend a frozen meal instead, they often will say, "Oh no, those meals are so high in salt." True, they are. But fast food isn't? Of course it is; we just don't see the grams of salt printed on the little box of fries, so we don't know how much salt is in them. Same goes for the fried chicken on our fast-food salads. I can tell you how much salt is in those meals: Way too much.

Diet soda is a drink I'll never really understand. I can see one or two a day. But like so many other things, it's gotten out of control. Many of us drink diet soda all day long. Diet drinks can be better than regular soda because they don't raise blood sugar and because they don't have calories. But there is nothing healthy about them. My friend refers to diet soda as a "can-o'-chemicals." Why are we OK with drinking super-mega-doses of artificial sodas but we can't eat a baked potato? And don't get me started on carrots. If you've ever read a diet book that tells you to stay away from carrots because they're too high in sugar, please think about that for a minute. Do you honestly think that eating too many carrots is contributing to the obesity problem in this country? And how can anyone sit there munching on their pork rinds and tell me that they won't eat carrots because they're too sugary? Question some of these outrageous behaviors before you adapt them into your lifestyle. Look at the whole forest, not just one tree.

All talk but no action: Remember my story about my tight pajamas and busy social calendar back in Chapter 1? Promising yourself that you'll start your new way of living a year from now, a month from now, or a week from now is just not good enough. If you're ready to feel healthier in body and spirit and happier about yourself, then it's time to start now. There will never be a perfect time to start. Your life will continue to be hectic and rushed. Ponder how you will get in better shape, but ponder it while taking a walk. There is a need for balance in this part of our lives, too. We can make graphs and charts and plan a weight-loss program until we're blue in the face, but if we don't start taking action, the plans mean nothing.

All action, no talk: If we don't have a road map (or a GPS), we'll have no idea where we're going. Our tactics will not work efficiently or effectively in the long run. For one thing, we can't continue moving forward without a plan. This is where we can fall prey to fooling ourselves. We think that we're working out more than we are or eating healthier than we are. Ninety percent of clients that I see come into my office with a week's food diary and as they hand it to me they say, "This week was really unusual; I didn't exercise or eat really well this week." Then, I ask how often they eat out, and I may hear one to two times per week. We look closely at the food diary and find out they actually ate out six out of seven days. Sometimes twice a day.

With no plan, we don't get good results because we aren't aware of what we're really doing. Instead, we're more aware of what we wish we were doing. So, write out your plan, or tell it to a friend. And then keep track of your actions.

Going to extremes. "I'll just stop eating." "I'll exercise six hours a day." "I will never eat chocolate again, for as long as I live." These are unrealistic, impossible-to-sustain concepts. Going from 0 to 60 is for Volkswagens, not humans. I hear people tell me that they were so successful when they were on a no-carb diet or when they exercised every day of the week. But the success was short-lived. So was it really successful? Long-term success is what we're looking for. And that means not going to such extremes that it becomes impossible to continue for any significant length of time.

Mistaking emotional hunger for physical hunger: We seem to use food as the answer to everything. We're giving food way too much credit by hoping that it satisfies our every need. What food can satisfy is physical hunger, and it can give us enjoyment along the way. What it can't do is … anything else. But many of us have decided that for whatever problem we have, food is the solution.

- When you've had a hard day, do you want to console yourself with comfort food?
- When something great has happened, do you want to celebrate with a treat?
- When you're sad or depressed, do you reach for the ice cream?
- When you're bored or procrastinating, do you start rummaging through your kitchen cabinets?

When food is what you do to manage feelings, you are an emotional eater. Through my own personal experience and my work as a nutrition counselor, I know a fair amount about this subject. But I wanted to consult an expert for this book. So I called Deb Elkin, a licensed professional counselor who specializes in "disordered eating," as she calls it. This is what she said: "When we feel bad, many of us use food to soothe or distract ourselves. If we're not willing to feel our feelings or don't know what they are because we're not in tune with them, we try to numb them with food."

According to research published in the International Journal of Obesity in 2003, many people fail to achieve weight goals when eating is used to regulate mood.[7]

"Something doesn't feel right. Am I lonely, tired, sad, afraid? Wait a minute; I think I'm just hungry. Yeah, that's it." When we mistake emotions for hunger, it may go something like this:
- Lonely = cheeseburger with fries
- Tired = ice cream with chocolate sauce
- Sad = cookies with milk
- Afraid = chimichanga with cheese

Believing that feeling tired equals failure: I am woman, hear me snore. We all try to do too much, men and women, but beating ourselves up because we're exhausted is particularly a bad emotional habit of women. ("I can bring home the bacon, fry it up in a pan. ...") Not only are we eating foods that zap our energy, but also we just keep going and going, and when we feel tired, we question our worth. And God forbid, if we ask for help, that would mean we're failures, right?

Sometimes, what we need is a nap. Or more nutritious food. Or, probably, both. So try not to get caught up in the cycle of feeling bad about being tired, then comforting yourself with junk food. Speaking of which ...

Using food as a reward: You had a bad day, a stressful day, or you met a deadline, had a good workout, got through your to-do list. You name it, and we reward ourselves with food. And this habit starts young. How many of us were potty trained with M&Ms? In grade school, I remember, if we did well on a test, we got a Coke.

"Food becomes a reward when you don't have a healthier reward system in place," says Elkin. "It's not OK to use food as a reward when it becomes a problem for you." For example:

- When it's the only reward you have.
- When you can't stop gaining weight.
- When you feel guilty about it.
- When you feel out of control.
- When you can't manage it.
- When you do it unconsciously.

"If you feel that food is the only thing that will make you feel better, you need to find other things to make you feel better," Elkin says.

The last-supper syndrome: You're at a party, and out comes the birthday cake. It's beautiful, and it looks very chocolatey. Sure, you've had chocolate cake before, but not THIS cake. Once it's gone, it's gone for good! You think, "I'd better grab a piece now, or I'll never know what I missed."

You have had chocolate cake before; you'll have it again. And it's OK to try a little piece now, if you can account for it in your total for the day.

Have you ever shopped for a car or house? It's easy to get caught up in the moment, and salespeople generally encourage that sort of emotion, too. You forget that even if this car or house is out of your price range, that one that DOES fit with your financial plan will come along soon enough — and you may like it even more than the one you're looking at right now. The same goes with diet plans, and chocolate cakes.

Falling for evil marketing: "It's only satisfying if you eat it," the Snickers slogan went. The Snickers people imply that the only way we can be satisfied is with their product. "With Betty Crocker Warm Delights, you're just three minutes away from heaven!" Who knew? All it takes to get to heaven is a microwave.

"Need a moment? Chew things over with Twix." Instead of sleeping on it, now we're chewing things over. "My moment. My Dove." If we want to do something nice for ourselves, we should have a candy bar. These marketers are using our weaknesses against us. And it's working.

And here are a few physical bad habits that stem from faulty reasoning:

Binge eating: If your child wanted a brownie, would you give him one, then another and another, until you're dishing out half the pan for him? Of course you wouldn't do that; it wouldn't be good for him. So why is it OK to do that to yourself? You've got to say no to yourself sometimes. Give yourself some boundaries. You know you want them.

Food inhalation: Most of us have perfectly good teeth. We just forget about them and inhale food so fast before we have time to enjoy it or chew it. This is acid reflux waiting to happen. And the quickest way to gain weight. You'll have missed out on the pleasure of eating because you didn't pay attention to it while it was happening. Have you ever looked down at your plate and your food was gone, and you can't remember eating it? Ouch.

Daily starvation routine: We have a mind-set of, "The longer I can go without eating, the better." So we try to hold out as long as possible. But as the day goes on, it becomes impossible. If we start the day out hungry, we'll tend to rev up our eating instead of wind down throughout the day. And then the vicious cycle of night eating begins. After eating late into the night, we try to hold out again the next day, deciding we won't eat much, and it slowly builds again. We get mad at ourselves for lack of "willpower." Stop the madness!

Where's the R-E-S-P-E-C-T?

Calling all women, and some men, too. We've got to stop putting ourselves last. After everyone else is fed, we'll take the scraps. After everything else is done, we'll take a tiny moment for ourselves and then feel guilty about it.

What are we, chopped liver? (A little high in cholesterol but a good source of iron.)

"Somewhere along the line, many of us were taught to not value ourselves; now, we need to learn to love ourselves," Elkin says.

It's time to learn how to love ourselves. Let's stop the negative patterns now. If we can recognize some of the stinkin' thinkin' that's been keeping us from reaching our goals, we can stop sabotaging ourselves and get our lives back where we want them. And our bodies, too.

Worksheet: Bad Habits

Review the self-defeating habits of thought listed in this chapter. Which ones are "inside of you"?
1. Being too hard on yourself.
2. Being too easy on yourself.
3. Assuming that getting older means getting out of shape.
4. Missing the forest for the trees.
5. All talk, no action.
6. All action, no talk.
7. Going to extremes.
8. Mistaking emotional hunger for physical hunger.
9. Believing that feeling tired equals failure.
10. Using food as a reward.
11. The last supper syndrome.
12. Falling for evil marketing.

Are there other negative thought patterns that are keeping you from achieving your goals?

_____

_____

_____

_____

Review the bad habits that stem from faulting reasoning. Do you do any of these?
1. Binge eating
2. Food inhalation
3. Daily starvation

Do you have other bad eating habits that come from your negative thought patterns listed above?

_____

_____

_____

_____

_____

Chapter 5

PFD to the Rescue

If I hear another health care professional say, "Get plenty of rest, eat right and exercise" ever again, I'll scream. For as long as I can remember, this recommendation has been the cornerstone of good health. Isn't it just stating the obvious? Is there really anyone alive who is unaware that getting plenty of rest, eating right and exercising is good for them?

The obesity epidemic is a complex issue. Oversimplified recommendations can be frustrating, ineffective and an insult to our intelligence. During nutrition consults, my weight loss clients oftentimes are overcome with emotion. It is not uncommon for them to break down and cry right there in my office. For years my response was to hand them a Kleenex. Eventually, I realized they don't need a soft tissue; they need a practical daily tool. They need to know *how* to fit plenty of rest, eating right and exercise into their lives. And so the Personal Food-tracking Device (PFD) was born.

What is it?

What exactly is a PFD (www.lifepreserverdiet.com), and why is it part of the Life Preserver Diet?

A PFD is a personal flotation device — a life preserver — and, in this case, a personal food-tracking device. Research shows that if people keep track of what they eat, they are better able

to maintain a healthy weight.[8] Why? Because you can see
what you're doing wrong and take corrective action. But to tell
someone to "keep track of what you eat" is a lot like saying,
"get plenty of rest, eat right and exercise." It sounds simple but
is actually very complicated. Keeping track of what you eat is
really a three-step process. First, you collect data by writing down
everything you eat, all day, every day. Once you have this data,
you must interpret the results: What are you eating too much
or too little of, where should you cut back, and what nutrients
are you missing? From there you must conclude how to apply
this information each and every day to your food choices. It's
time consuming, and it can take the enjoyment
out of eating. With this little PFD you
reap all the benefits of this three-step
process without having to do the work
yourself. It keeps track of what you
eat, counts your calories, makes sure
you get all of the nutrients that you
need and not too much of what you
don't need. It's your personal little
life preserver. If you feel like you're in
too deep, now you can get your head
above water.

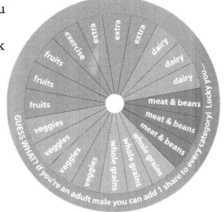

Who designed the PFD? You and me together.
I created this with the help of all my clients. I listened to people
like you and came up with several versions. The one that stuck
was the one that showed the most results and helped people get to
and maintain a healthy weight. The PFD is based on the USDA's
MyPlate (the guidelines formerly known as the food pyramid)
and the dietary guidelines for Americans, which are designed to
promote optimal nutrition and prevent disease.

What the PFD does

A basic truth: When you don't pay attention to what you eat, you won't ever know whether you're "eating right," whatever that is. But who wants to keep a complicated diary?

Here's what a typical day might look like for a gal on the go:
- Breakfast — sesame bagel & cream cheese
- Lunch — flour tortilla with black beans and cheese
- Dinner — pizza with cheese and pepperoni
- Snack — popcorn

It doesn't look all that bad, but maybe we should look closer. What food groups were eaten in this day? Mostly white breads and cheese. Not one fruit or vegetable.

Another day falls short:
- Breakfast — Cereal and milk
- Snack — Peanut butter crackers
- Lunch — Chicken sandwich, fries and a salad
- Snack — M&Ms
- Dinner — Pasta with garlic bread and broccoli
- Dessert — Ice cream

This day has a couple of vegetables thrown in, but it's still way too heavy on the carbs.

Your PFD turns that vague "eat right" advice into specific guidelines by doing three things: It keeps you on a food "budget;" it simplifies meal planning, and it focuses your decision-making.

Your food budget: Staying within limits

Eating right is like living on a budget. You've got to pay attention to where all the nickels and dimes go, and you've got to pay attention to where all those little calories go, too. A pair of shoes here, a candy bar there ... you don't think you're spending much, or eating much, but somehow it all adds up.

I'm pretty good at keeping track of what I eat, but when it comes to money ... not so much. If I've got money in my wallet, then I tend to spend it — regardless of whether I've paid my bills this month. I don't think much about it. But at the end of the day, I look in my wallet and find nothing left. I don't really know where the money went. I didn't think I was spending that much.

For some people, it's the same thing with eating. They don't think about it. They might "spend" an entire day's worth of calories on a pint of Ben & Jerry's Chubby Hubby ice cream (1,320), or on a Burger King Double Whopper with cheese (1,060). But it doesn't seem like they ate all that much ... they even skipped the fries!

I have had some frustrating conversations on the phone with my credit union when my monthly statement shows that I have overdrawn charges yet again. Those charges sneak up on me. They come out of nowhere. Apparently, I need a better system to keep track of my money. The PFD will be the system *you* need to help you stay on track with your food "budget." No more pounds that sneak in without you knowing what happened. You are in control now.

That's not all the PFD can do. Your little life preserver doesn't stop there. It not only simplifies your food budget, but it also simplifies meal-planning and decision-making.

Meal-planning: When you have too much on your plate, you'll gain weight

When we're in a time crunch, exercising and eating healthily are often the first things to go. We put them off until our bones get weak, our clothes don't fit and we feel like strangers in our own bodies. Then it feels hopeless. Who has time to squeeze in some exercise or plan what to eat? Even as a nutritionist — for whom food is supposed to be at the forefront of my mind — I am often guilty of not planning my meals. There are many days when I know that I'm going to be gone for 12 hours and I've got no food with me, no food where I'm going and no food plan. Just money that I'll spend that day on whatever is easy to grab.

On most days, I feel like I'm doing good to just get to work on time. By 9 a.m. I've rushed to get out of my house, fought traffic, snagged a parking spot … and I'm already stressed as I walk through my office door. Then I look at my daunting To Do list. There's nobody running to my rescue because like me, everyone has too much to do. We're all in the same boat — overwhelmed with responsibility. The PFD is a tool designed to share the burden and come to your rescue, making it easier for you to eat healthily. It makes meal planning so simple. The PFD will make meal planning easier by helping you know what to shop for and what to have at home. Use it when planning menus for the week and when making grocery lists. The new National Heart, Lung, and Blood Institute Obesity Guidelines say that you can reduce the time you spend cooking healthy meals by using a shopping list and keeping a well-stocked kitchen.[9]

Now, you will have one less thing on your plate.

Decision-making: Make it easy on yourself

"I could lose weight if you tell me exactly what to eat every day. There are too many choices out there." Most of my clients say that to me at some point. Have you ever gone to the grocery store to grab something for dinner, thinking you'll decide what to get once you're there, but then, for the life of you, can't figure out what to get? You go up and down the aisles just waiting for something to jump out at you. Too many choices can be overwhelming and complicated. Less is more when it comes to making food choices. The PFD will help simplify your life. Decision-making will be much easier. Go ahead, now's a good time to let out a sigh of relief. From now on, as you go through the day, your little PFD will tell you what's left on the menu. No share, beware (more on food shares later) … until tomorrow when you start all over again. You are on a permanent vacation from trying to figure out what to eat each day. And who doesn't love a vacation?

Why it works

What is the philosophy behind the PFD? The U.S. Department of Agriculture's MyPlate is based on variety, moderation and balance. And so is the PFD. But there's also science behind its simple system.

Variety: Keep it interesting; eat from all food groups

Carbohydrates increase body fat
Carbohydrates decrease body fat
Fat is healthy

Fat is unhealthy
Eat more protein
Eat less protein
Eat more chicken
Eat less chicken
Soy decreases cancer risk
Soy increases cancer risk

The science behind nutrition recommendations is ever-changing. We are always learning more! Also, each food offers its own unique nutrients. So the safest, healthiest (and tastiest) approach is to mix it up. Have a little bit of everything and not too much of anything. And when in doubt, eat the simpler, fresher choice: a whole apple instead of a package of apple chips; grilled or roasted instead of battered and fried; a big salad instead of a frozen dinner.

Moderation: Enjoy, but don't overdo it

"Do not eat cookies. No more cookies. Cookies are bad." If this is what you are thinking, what will be in the back of your mind all day? "I want cookies. Why can't I have cookies? I wish I could eat cookies. Everybody else eats cookies."

My advice: Please have a cookie … and move on. Clear the space in your brain for other thoughts. Just don't eat five cookies; have one or two. And the next day, have one or two again. Cutting out foods, even cookies, can be detrimental to your well-being. There are no bad foods. All foods fit. We just need for the majority of our food choices to be healthy. Besides, when we incorporate all of the food groups into our diets, there really isn't much room to overdo it on extras.

Balance and proportion: Eat more of some food groups than others

Here's a big one, something we are forever trying to achieve. Just when we thought we had balance in our lives, something gets out of whack. We can be doing great at work, but things at home aren't going so smoothly. Or we can be spending a lot of time with family, but our finances are messed up. Right now, do this exercise, please. Stand up, lift up one leg at the knee, and point your toe. Go ahead, try it for 30 seconds. If you start falling to the left, you need to lean to the right. And visa versa. It's a constant adjustment. Balancing is dynamic. In order to achieve balance we need to pay attention to which way we're falling, so we can adjust properly. The Dietary Guidelines for Americans emphasizes more fruits, vegetables, whole grains, low fat milk products, lean protein, beans, eggs and nuts and less saturated fat, trans fats, cholesterol, salt and sugar. Your PFD is designed to help you keep that proportion intact on a daily basis. If you use it to guide your choices consistently, you will automatically achieve a healthy balance of the desired nutrients that your body needs.

OK, you can sit down now.

The science: Let's talk calories

There are several equations used to estimate calorie needs: Harris-Benedict, Mifflin-St. Jeor, kcalories per kilogram of body weight and USDA's MyPlate are some used by registered dietitians. These are all estimates on calorie needs. Individual needs vary and must be adjusted based on your results. ChooseMyPlate. gov offers charts on calorie needs depending on age, gender and activity level. On first glance the calorie needs appear higher than when using some of the other formulas. But the calories you see on the chart are for weight *maintenance*. In order to lose one pound per week, you'd need to decrease the calories by 500 per day. So if you fall under a 2,000 calorie a day recommendation for weight maintenance on MyPlate and want to lose weight, you'd need to eat 1,500 calories per day. The PFD is based on a diet of approximately 1,500 to 1,700 calories per day, which is appropriate for most women age 19 years and older (discretionary calories are included in estimations in food groups). Each share is approximately 100 calories (300 calories for a whole food group) except for vegetables and fruit, which are 50 calories per share. Once you're at a desirable body weight, you'll want to experiment with increasing calorie amounts. And if you're one of the unfortunate people who require fewer than 2,000 calories a day to maintain weight, you may need to experiment with reducing your serving sizes to reach your desired weight.

How you do it

The big picture

- By logging in, you always have access to this little life preserver that contains your meal plan.
- You eat.
- You mark off what you ate. (You eat fruit, you mark a fruit share; you eat meat, you mark a meat share. We'll talk about share sizes later.)
- You meet your nutrient needs for the day.
- You eat low-fat, low-calorie, high-fiber foods without having to think much about it.
- At the end of day, you feel nourished and energized with a sense of accomplishment.

The details

3 shares whole grains
3 shares meat & beans
3 shares fruit
1 share exercise

3 shares dairy
4 shares veggies
3 shares extra

Whole grains

- What they provide: Magnesium, thiamin, fiber, folate and iron.
- Foods included in whole grain category: Anything made mostly of whole grains: amaranth, barley, buckwheat, bulgur, graham flour, millet, wheat berries, whole grain corn, whole kamut, whole oats, whole rye, whole spelt and whole wheat. (Look for the phrase "100 percent whole wheat" on packaging)
- A share is approximately: 100 calories
- A share looks like:
  1/2 cup cooked brown rice
  1/2 cup cooked whole wheat pasta
  1/2 cup cooked quinoa
  1 small corn tortilla
  1 medium slice seven-grain bread
  2 cups microwave popcorn
  1 cup Cheerios
  6 Triscuits
- The bottom line: On average, a 100-calorie share is about 1/2 cup cooked grains. When in doubt, "one serving" as described on the package nutritional information is 1 share.

Dairy

- What they provide: Calcium, potassium, vitamin D and protein.
- Foods included in the dairy category: Milk, yogurt and cheese.
- A share is approximately 100 calories

- A share looks like:
    1 cup skim or 1 percent milk (or enriched soy milk)
    6 ounces (1 container) lowfat vanilla yogurt
        (or enriched soy yogurt)
    1/2 cup lowfat cottage cheese
    1 ounce (1 slice) cheddar cheese
- The bottom line: In general, the denser the dairy product, the smaller the share size. Milk gives you the largest serving size, at 1 cup for 1 share. What a deal!

Meat & beans
- What they provide: Vitamin B6, vitamin E, niacin, zinc, fiber and protein.
- Foods included in the meat and beans category: Meat (especially lean meats, such as poultry and fish), legumes such as beans or lentils, eggs, soy protein, peanut butter
- A share is approximately: 100 calories.
- A share looks like:
    3 slices lean deli meat
    1/2 small split chicken breast
    1/2 salmon steak
    1/2 small sirloin
    1 small lean pork chop
    1 veggie burger
    1 tablespoon peanut butter
    1/2 cup tofu
    1/2 cup black beans or chickpeas
    1/2 cup cooked lentils
    1 egg
- The bottom line: On average, a 100-calorie share weighs about 2 ounces. An appropriate dinner portion of meat counts as 2 shares; a lunch portion counts as 1 share.

Fruit
- What they provide: Vitamin A, vitamin C, potassium, fiber, folate and antioxidants.
- Foods included in the fruit category: Whole raw fruits, apple sauce, juices, all-fruit popsicles, dried fruit
- A share is approximately: 50 calories
- A share looks like:
  > 1 small apple
  > 1 small banana
  > 1/2 medium grapefruit
  > 1/2 cup orange juice
  > 1 slice melon
  > 1 cup berries
- The bottom line: On average, a 50-calorie share is a whole fruit. One small piece of fruit counts as 1 share. One-half cup juice or two tablespoons dried fruit counts as 1 share.

Vegetables
- What they provide: Vitamin A, vitamin C, potassium, iron, fiber and antioxidants.
- Foods included in the vegetable category: Nonstarchy and starchy vegetables (corn, potatoes and squash), raw dressed vegetables (salads), vegetable juice
- A share is approximately: 50 calories, including a small amount of fat that you may cook them in or add to them.
- A share looks like:
  > 1/2 cup cooked starchy veggies
  > 1 cup cooked nonstarchy veggies
  > 2 cups salad with 1 tablespoon dressing
  > 1 cup vegetable juice
  > Raw, undressed veggies are free —
  > > eat as many as you like!

- The bottom line: In general, vegetables fall into two categories: starchy (corn, peas, winter squash, potatoes) and nonstarchy (carrots, broccoli, spinach, mushrooms, summer squash). One share is about 1/2 cup cooked starchy or 1 cup cooked nonstarchy vegetables (including a small amount of fat for cooking), or 2 cups salad with 1 tablespoon dressing. Raw, undressed salads and vegetables are so low in calories, they don't even count as a share — you can eat an unlimited amount.

Extras
- Foods included in the extras category: Anything that doesn't fall into any of the other categories — any grains that aren't whole grains (the white stuff), sweets and snacks.
- A share is: Anything equaling approximately 100 calories.
- A share looks like:
  1 slice white bread
  1/2 cup white rice
  1/2 cup cooked white pasta
  1 small bag potato chips
  1/2 cup ice cream
  10 nut halves
  3 miniature peanut butter cups
  4 chocolate kisses
  Fried foods — Add one extra share to each share
       of fried meat or veggie
- Bottom line: You choose to use these extras any way that you'd like. Each "extra" share equals about 100 calories. Read labels to learn how many calories your favorite snack foods have. If you choose to use your extra shares for a few pieces of chocolate, ice cream, French fries, it's your choice. But choose carefully because 300 calories goes quickly. You may also use your extra shares for carry-over. For example, if you have no more whole

grain spaces for the day, but you eat another whole grain, it counts as an extra.

Exercise
There is a share for exercise on your PFD every day. That one share is just as important as the food shares. Any amount counts. It's OK to start out slow. You will pick up momentum as you go. (Check out Chapter 8.)

Get plenty of rest

An estimated 60 percent of American women say they only get a good night's sleep a few nights a week, according to the National Sleep Foundation. Researchers at the University of Chicago have found that partial sleep deprivation alters hormone levels that regulate hunger, causing an increase in appetite and a preference for calorie-dense food. (Dec 7, 2004, annals of Internal Medicine).[10] You've heard people brag about how little sleep they can function on. I've done it myself. As if somehow we're tougher if we can survive on less sleep. If we can just stay up a little longer, we can be so much more productive. We keep going and going like the little Energizer bunny. But, it may be detrimental to our weight loss goals and our health, not to mention our happiness. Who wants to be walking around tired and grumpy all the time? Be strict with yourself, like you would with a child at bedtime. Watch one less hour of TV at night. Do one less load of laundry; send one less e-mail. Log off of Facebook. When it's bedtime, it's lights out. You'll be so much happier, and so will the people around you.

A sample day using the PFD

Breakfast

You wake up and have 1 cup whole grain cereal (mark one share whole grains, and you have two left for the day).
1 cup milk (mark one dairy; two left)
1 banana (1 fruit; two left)

Lunchtime

You brought a ham and cheese sandwich on a whole-grain pita with three slices ham and 1 slice cheese (one whole grain, one left; one meat and beans, two left; one dairy, you have one left). (The sandwich has tomato slices and lettuce — those are free!) You have a small bag of chips with lunch (one extra share; two left) and 1 cup vegetable soup (one vegetable down — three left).

Afternoon snack

Three small pieces dark chocolate equaling 100 calories (one more extra left) one apple (one fruit left)

Dinner

Here's what we have left: three shares veggies, one whole grain, two shares meat & beans, one share dairy, one share fruit and one extra. How about 1 cup cooked brown rice (1 share whole grain plus one extra), 1/2 cup peas, 1 cup asparagus, 1 cup cauliflower, and 3 ounces sirloin, cut into strips? That sounds like a great stir-fry!

After dinner

A container of yogurt and 3/4 cup berries. (That was your last dairy and your last fruit for the day. You did it!)

"What if I get hungry?": Don't fret. If at any point in the day you get a little peckish, have a cup of tea with a teaspoon of honey. Go ahead. 20 calories won't hurt you. And you can always nosh on some raw veggies: red bell peppers, snow peas, green beans, cucumbers, radishes. (See ... I didn't even mention celery sticks!)

A note for men: You may have noticed that this book is directed, for the most part, at women. But that doesn't mean, dear sir, that the advice won't work for you, too. In fact, here's a bonus for you: Because men, generally speaking, are larger than women and have greater caloric needs, you get to eat more! Add an additional share to every category. Just don't rub it in.

PFD 101

Now that you know how it works, let it work for you! This little life preserver will keep you on your food budget, simplify meal planning, and help you make healthy food choices. You may want to refer back to this chapter and lists for guidance along the way. Your PFD is a practical, effective tool that will help you with the daily choices and planning that are essential to any healthy lifestyle. You no longer have to sit back and listen to empty advice like eat right, exercise and get plenty of rest. Instead of feeling angry, frustrated or overcome with emotion because of being unable to meet your weight goals, you can now rejoice. You won't just be hearing the mantra of "eat right, exercise and get plenty of rest" anymore. Now you'll be living it. You will walk the walk and have all the help you need every step of the way.

Now, just sign on the dotted line.

The Contract: A promise to yourself

I, _____ , agree to stay on the Life Preserver Diet for three months. I know that I will not be perfect, because nobody is. If I feel better, look better and get closer to my goal in that time, I will continue on this journey and renew my contract for three more months.

Signed: _____

Date: _____

Chapter 6

The Secret to Happiness ...
(A few thoughts on the importance of attitude)

Losing weight depends on a simple formula of burning more calories than you take in, but keeping weight off is based on something much, much deeper. It's about loving yourself enough to make big, sometimes difficult changes of habit. It's about putting yourself above all others, for at least a few minutes each day. It's about recognizing that it takes time and patience to learn new ways of doing things and to see the results of that effort.

Attitude IS important. An attitude of self-love. But loving yourself doesn't mean overfeeding yourself. It means taking care of your own health as well as you take care of the other members of your family. And that, of course, sometimes includes tough love. (Don't love yourself "enough" to feed yourself an ice cream sandwich. Love yourself even more, and say no!)

Closer to fine

If money and time were no object and you could live any life you wanted, what would it look like? For me, it would involve good music, good food, and lots of time with my family. But of course, there would have to be exercise (probably dancing the night away) to balance out the good food — because I'd want to have a fabulous figure to show off all those designer clothes I'd own.

How about you? Do you imagine yourself living the spa lifestyle? A hammock, a pool, a personal chef, a personal trainer, a personal shopper? Sounds good!

OK, when I count to three and snap my fingers; you're back to reality. Ready? One, two, three. Goodbye, personal chef! Goodbye, Giorgio the pool boy! But here's the point of this exercise: Even if you have limited time and limited money, you can still bring bits and pieces of this fantasy life into your real life — right now. Maybe you can't have a chef, but you can cook some tasty, healthful meals for yourself. Maybe you can't work out with a personal trainer every day, but you might be able to swing a one-on-one consultation with the exercise physiologist at your local Y or wellness center to get started on a workout routine.

Maybe you can't eat perfectly every day, and maybe you can't do a full workout every day. But remember that old Indigo Girls song? Anything you CAN do, every day, gets you "closer to fine."

Attitude is everything! And attitude has momentum. No one ever stays the same forever — you're always changing; you're always moving in one direction or the other. It's amazing how fast we can abandon our very best intentions. You can wake up one morning all ready to face a new day, and then a traffic jam makes you late for work, and you don't have time to go to the gym and … why bother? You might as well eat a bag of chips for dinner. THAT is the "why bother" attitude, and it drags you in the wrong direction.

Which direction are you headed? Are you getting happier, becoming more satisfied with who you are? Or are you moving in that OTHER direction?

Ask yourself: Are you getting closer to fine?

Turning it around

So now you know what your fantasy healthy lifestyle would be like. But how do you put those "closer to fine" ideas into practice each day?

You may not always make the right choices. But you know what? When you do one little thing for yourself, you get more confident. And then the next little thing that you do for yourself seems that much easier.

When it's 10 in the morning and your co-worker stops by your desk with a box of doughnuts, you need to be armed with self-love and a long-term perspective in order to keep your hands at your sides. So let's look at some of the ways you can turn those negative thoughts into a positive attitude.

• **Start every day with an emotional check-in.** When you greet your friends you ask them, "How are you?" When's the last time you asked yourself that? Start each day with a, "How am I?" Are you feeling powerful and ready to tackle whatever life throws at you? Are you feeling a little down? If this is feeling like a power day, then you're good to go. You laugh in the face of doughnuts! But if you're feeling kinda vulnerable, then steel yourself for what's ahead. Remind yourself of where you're going. If you felt down when you looked in the mirror, remind yourself that a day is coming, very soon, when your favorite clothes look great again. Remind yourself of that when those doughnuts come a-calling.

- **Remember that your plate is half full, not half empty.** You're not depriving yourself when you limit your portions, but you are depriving yourself when you eat more than you should: depriving yourself of feeling and looking your best.

- **Get a "used-to" makeover.** I can't tell you how many times my new clients start their nutrition counseling sessions with "I used to …": "I used to be so fit." "I used to wear a size 6." "I used to be able to eat whatever I wanted and never gain weight." They spend their time thinking of where they used to be and feeling bad about where they are now. But before you can get back to a happier, healthier you, you need to accept where you are now. Guess what? Everyone in their early 20s can eat whatever they want! But by the time you reach your 40s, it doesn't work that way.

  The thing to do is spin those "used-tos" forward, to the present. Stop pining for the old you; celebrate the used-tos that you can discard. Indulge in a new behavior. Turn the "I used to" phrase into something new and positive. So instead of saying, "I used to be able to run up two flights of stairs," now say, "I used to take the elevator; now I use the stairs at work." I used to eat a lot of junk food; now I love fresh veggies! I used to break into a sweat carrying groceries from my car; now I can walk twice around my block! Introduce yourself to the new you; reinvent yourself. The person who used to need instant gratification of food as a reward is gone.

- **Remember the true goal is well-being.** You'll feel better not when you reach a certain size but when the excess on your body is really gone. The reward is in feeling better, being more fit. Looking great is the gravy!

- **Recalibrate your satisfaction meter.** Think of eating until you feel nourished, not until you feel stuffed and uncomfortable.

Managing time

"Who has time to exercise?" "Who has time to cook?" I have been asked these questions hundreds, perhaps thousands, of times by clients. And my answer is always the same: You do! You might have to make a few adjustments to your schedule, but trust me, we're not talking about a LOT of time here, and besides, you're worth it!

The secret is time management — about choosing priorities. You DO have just 30 minutes in your day to go on a walk or to exercise with a DVD or to just dance in your living room with the radio turned up. And you DO have time to cook a few simple meals a week. But first, you have to get rid of something that's secretly eating up some time during your busy day.

Let me give you an example. I love "Modern Family." It's just 30 minutes every week that I really enjoy. But often, once the show is over, I continue to sit. Usually I'm indifferent to whatever show ABC has put in the lineup in the next slot, but unless I tell myself before I turn on the TV that it's going off again as soon as my half-hour is up, I usually sit through that next show, anyway.

There's a half-hour, right there, when I could be hula hooping! For that matter, if I were really short on time, I could hula hoop while I'm watching "Modern Family" and not miss a single line. A twist for every plot twist, so to speak.

Here's another example. I know how crazy dinner time is; I'm sure yours is, too. But how much time do I waste waiting in a drive-through line after work? It doesn't really take any longer to make a simple, fresh dinner than the typical wait time for a take-out dinner order. The time is there; it's just hidden in our schedules.

Most of us women are programmed to give and give. We don't even realize sometimes how much of our day is devoted to others. But every once in a while, we lose it! We get angry and resentful because we feel like we've lost ourselves amid all the things we do for everyone else. We never get to be "selfish" and do something just for ourselves. Well, I'm here to tell you: It's not selfish to take care of yourself, to even do something nice for yourself. It helps us feel good about taking care of all the other people we love.

We're not asking for much here. We're not asking to be ladies of leisure. We're only asking for a little bit of time, just for ourselves. You can be rippin' and runnin' all day from the minute you wake up until the moment you go to bed. But no matter what else happens in your day, as long as when your head hits the pillow you can say that you exercised and you stuck with your eating plan, that's when your time has been managed. You got your workout in and you didn't stuff yourself — you've been livin' the life preserver life.

Expect chaos

We all know what mornings are like. At my house, the morning involves getting my child up, dressed, fed and out the door in time for the school bus while still conducting my early-morning business (e-mails and phone calls, most days) and getting myself showered, dressed, fed and out the door. If I leave 15 minutes too late, I add at least a half-hour to my commute. So time is of the essence.

While all that is going on, can I really expect to make a lunch for myself, too? That simply is NOT going to happen — at least not until they perfect that cloning thing.

My only solution is to plan for the chaos. Since I know I will simply never find the time to make a sandwich in the morning, I have to plan ahead … but just by a few hours. Sometimes, that sandwich — or packing a few leftovers — is the last thing I do before I go to bed. But it's worth it because I know that if I don't, I will be eating some processed, salty, fatty, flavorless fast food for lunch.

Managing critics

Critics come in all forms. Some are casual contacts, like the dieting co-worker who raises an eyebrow when you enjoy your after-lunch chocolate mint. And some are more vocal and destructive, even if they don't mean to be. These critics might even live with you.

Let's say that you've announced to your spouse that you've decided to make some changes in your life for the better. Your loved one may be very proud of you. But when those changes start affecting your regular routine (and the family's), don't be surprised if you catch some static.

For example, perhaps for many years, the two of you have

watched TV after dinner. But now, you want to get in a short walk every night. This may not appeal to your spouse.

"Hey, where are you going, Miss Walks-Every-Night? We've got 'CSI' to watch!"

Don't let anyone stop you. Don't let anything stop you. Prove your doubters wrong. Everyone thinks their diet and exercise plan is the best, and just about everyone wants to tell you all about it. And hey, their plan probably is best … for them. But you now have a vision of what is best for you and what you're going to do to get there. So stick with it.

Worksheet: Happiness Planner

What can you do to create and maintain a positive attitude? Identify some of your personal "optimism obstacles" — does your tight wardrobe depress you? Do trusted friends doubt your will? Does exhaustion weaken your spirit? Then write down what you can do to turn that frown upside down.

Tight wardrobe   I'm going to get into that little black dress soon!

Doubting friend   If she wants to join me on my lunchtime walk, she can.

Too tired to cook   I can make a pot of chili on Sundays.

Downers	New attitude
1._____	_____
2._____	_____
3._____	_____
4._____	_____
5._____	_____

Chapter 7

The Secret to Eating:
A little bit every day

You now know what an important role attitude plays in meeting your goals. You're mentally prepared and ready to get down to the nitty-gritty of healthy eating. This chapter will guide you, step by step, through the three phases of the Life Preserver Diet.

There is an art to eating healthfully for a lifetime. Any amateur "dieter" can eat healthily for a little while — depriving themselves and being miserable. But it takes a visionary with creativity and passion to make it stick for the long haul. A lifelong change needs to be simple yet enjoyable. It takes perseverance and a sense of adventure to make it through the tough times.

You're no tourist! You're a world traveler ready to discover what lies ahead. So let's get moving.

Think of the next several weeks of your life as falling into three phases:

Phase 1: Charting your course. This is the planning process where you get your provisions in place. This process is meant to be fun, a way to bring out your own flair and surround yourself with some simple pleasures.

Phase 2: Anchor's away. You put the PFD to use and learn the do's and don'ts of good eating.

Phase 3: Smooth sailing. You focus on your mind-set while you enjoy the trip.

Phase 1: Charting your course

This phase gets us prepared for the journey ahead. We'll take a close look at the step-by-step process of meal planning. A 2006 study published in The International Journal of Behavioral Nutrition and Physical Activity found that people who plan meals ahead of time tend to be more successful at weight loss and weight maintenance.[11] If we don't plan for ourselves, it's easy to fall victim to someone else's plan for us. We become part of McDonald's and KFC's plan. In fact, they are banking on our not having a plan.

Getting all of your supplies in place may take a few days or a week. It's OK. You're taking critical steps here.

First, decide where you spend most of your time — at home, the office, your car, hotels? Preparing for the days ahead doesn't only mean preparing for meals at home. It means stocking up in the places where you spend your time. That way you don't have to eat so many meals out.

The workplace stash

If you work away from home, then you probably eat meals (and snacks) there on a regular basis. Except, you can do better than making a meal out of a candy bar from the vending machine. Instead, stock up on real plates and bowls (they brighten your day and make paper-sack meals seem more substantial), forks, knives, spoons, and some plastic resealable bags.

In addition, keep a small stash of easy-to-prepare foods in a desk drawer or cabinet. Here are some foods to consider:

Whole grains
- Whole grain crackers: Reduced-fat Wheat Thins or Triscuits go well with anything.
- Dry cereal: Individually packaged or in a full-size box. Look for about 5 grams of fiber and 5 grams of protein per serving. (5/5)
- Instant whole-grain hot cereals in individual packets, such as oatmeal or Kashi Golean brand cereals.
- Whole grain bread: Try rye, whole wheat or seven-grain.

If you have access to a refrigerator and microwave, add these items to your list:
- Whole grain frozen waffles
- Popcorn: Mini bags, lightly buttered if you must.

Fruits
- Fresh: Apples, bananas and oranges will store well for a few days at room temperature.
- Vacuum sealed or canned: Packaged fruit cups and individual servings of unsweetened apple sauce will keep indefinitely.
- Dried: Choose fruits without added sugar, and watch those serving sizes! A few raisins or dried apricots can add up to lots of calories quickly (1 share is 1/4 cup).

If you have access to a refrigerator, add:
- Any fresh fruit: Try some exotic additions such as Asian pears, kiwi, mango, persimmons. Experiment with what's in season. Berries are great to have around — add them to yogurt or cereal.

Dairy
- If you don't have a refrigerator, you can keep on hand a few individual serving-size boxes of vacuum-packed, ultrapasteurized milk. Enjoy a midday cereal break or just drink some milk on the rocks in place of a soda. Fortified soy milk is packed in individual-size drink boxes, too.

If you have access to a refrigerator, add:
- Cheese: Individually packed servings are convenient and stay fresh longer.
- Yogurt: Nonfat or lowfat is a good choice.
- Milk: Skim or 1 percent, organic (nonhomogenized if you can find it; it's better for you)
- Cottage cheese: The small individual containers are the perfect size.

Vegetables
- Fresh broccoli florets, raw green beans and carrots will last a day or two at your desk.

If you have access to a refrigerator, add:
- Prewashed salad greens as well as fresh, cut-up bell peppers (red, yellow, orange, green), cucumbers, celery and cauliflower to your list.

If you have access to a freezer and a microwave, add:
- Frozen veggies. Green Giant Steamers can be a whole meal!

Meat & beans
- Peanut butter: Good on bananas, apples, crackers, waffles and almost anything. But watch your serving size (1 tablespoon is a share).

- Chicken or tuna: Choose the vacuum-packed individual serving sizes for easy storage. Tuna packed in water instead of oil has less fat. A recent report concluded that "light" tuna often has less mercury than the more expensive Albacore variety.
- Canned beans: Keep a few small cans of chickpeas or black beans around. You can dump them on a green salad for a serving of protein or just eat them with a fork for a hearty snack.

If you have access to a refrigerator, add:
- Hummus: Great with carrot sticks, whole wheat bread or pretzels.
- Deli meats: Boars Head products are less processed than most.

Extras
- "Energy" bars and other individually packed snacks — try to stick with the 5/5 rule (roughly 5 grams of fiber and 5 grams of protein), and about 100 calories per "extra" share.
- Beverages: Flavored carbonated waters feel like a soda, without all the artificial sweeteners. No shares!

The car stash
According to a 2008 study done by the U.S. Department of Agriculture Economic Research Service, when people have long intervals between meals, they are likely to consume more calories when they do eat a meal.[12] Eating smaller amounts more often will keep you from overeating at mealtime. If you have a little something to hold you over until you get home, you'll eat less when you get there and make better choices — you won't be starving by the time you walk in the door. I try to eat a snack in the car that is good for me and that I don't eat much of otherwise. I'm stuck there, so I might as well make the best of it.

Obviously, many foods can't be kept in the car, but you may want to keep it simple and just grab something from your office stash to eat on your way home. For commuters with a long drive and lots of traffic, you may need to upgrade from Car Stash to Road Rage Prevention Kit. The kit could include audio books, favorite tunes and a stress ball in addition to the healthy snacks.

Drawing the map

Once you have your stashes in place, you are ready to plan your weekly menu.

1. Look at the calendar for the week ahead. Decide which nights you'll have time to cook. Shoot for two or three nights per week. The other nights you can eat leftovers or simple throw-together recipes. (See Chapter 10). You may be tempted to start planning elaborate nightly dinners. But try to keep your plan realistic. Remember, we want to simplify our lives.

2. Pick two or three dinners to cook and two or three throw-together meals. Use your PFD to help you get in all of your food groups.

Things to keep in mind while you're creating weekly menus:

- **Give yourself** permission to cook even if you're not a gourmet. Like everything else, you'll get better with practice.

- **Think about** eating a little meat with your veggies, not a few veggies with your meat.

- **Step away** from the diet food. It's less satisfying than the real stuff, and it's only low-calorie if you eat small amounts. Get back to more whole foods that are rich in flavor and nutrients.

- **Enjoy** the process. Have fun with it.

  - Create a dinner menu for the week, and display it in the kitchen. Give your kids creative license to style it with markers and stickers, or buy a white board and display daily specials, restaurant style.

  - Now go back to your calendar and pick the days that you'll be eating lunch at home, in the office and at a restaurant. If you notice that you eat lunch out most days, start planning to bring your lunch to work more often. Reverse the trend: Eat in most days and out on some.

  - If it helps you plan, make a lunch menu and display it in the kitchen. Or, you may just want to buy a variety of lunch foods and wait until the night before to decide what to have. (This goes for kids' lunches also.) Use your PFD to help you select lunch items.

Now, you've got your weekly menus planned and displayed. It feels good, doesn't it?

  - Make a grocery list. Use your menus to make your list and add breakfast and snack items, including sweets.

  - Don't forget a Candy Plan! I have a confession to make. I eat chocolate almost every morning. My favorite is Ghirardelli dark. I don't recommend this for everyone, but it works for me — and the Candy Plan has worked for many of my clients. I used to try to stay away from chocolate completely because it was the one sweet that I couldn't eat just a little of. I would go for weeks without any chocolate at all. Then, when my guard was down, I'd have one small piece … and another and another. I couldn't stop. I'd feel horrible and swear off chocolate again. It was a vicious cycle. I was complaining about this to my sister one day. She said, "Why don't you just eat a little bit every day?" It sounded ludicrous to me because I had never eaten just a little chocolate. But I tried it, and I liked it. I can stop after a bite or two, because I know the next morning I can jump out of bed and have more Ghirardelli. The idea of eating chocolate every day and not feeling guilty about it — wow. Now I eat 100 calories of chocolate every day and use it as one of my PFD extras. It helps that they're wrapped in single servings. Life is good.

Do what works for you. Maybe you need a Cookie Plan or a Twinkie Plan.

Time to go shopping

I love this part. Grocery shopping is my idea of fun. I probably need to get out more.

But still, when I have my list, I can sashay through the store with such ease, not worrying about what to get because I've got my list. Sure, I'll grab one or two impulse items, but for the most part I stick to the list.

My favorite part of buying groceries is at the checkout counter. I don't know if anyone else does this or if I'm just a freak, but I take great pride in my grocery cart. When I'm at the checkout line I admire my items as I place them on the conveyer belt. I enjoy seeing all the colors of the fresh produce, the textures of the grains and richness of the dairy. I group them in lovely little cornucopia bundles as they roll by the cashier, so I can relish in their beauty. I feel like the Vincent Van Gogh of grocery shopping. What a beautiful still-life painting I've created, right here at Publix on a Sunday afternoon! I feel satisfied that I'm doing something good for me and my family. (And I try not to smirk at the people around me, with their junk food and fried chicken and instant dinners.)

Try it the next time you're at the grocery store. Build your own still life at the check out counter. Just don't take too long and make enemies with the people in the line behind you.

OK, your meals are planned, and your fridge is stocked with fresh, fragrant, wholesome foods. You've made thoughtful choices of what goes in your refrigerator and pantry. It wasn't a forced, desperate decision, made while rushing on a weeknight, unprepared. By Sunday evening you're ready for the week. You are Superwoman. You are an artiste.

Set aside a day each week to chart your course for the next week. Get in the new habit of planning every week. The time you spend planning in the beginning of the week will save you many wasted hours, standing confused in a grocery store aisle or, even worse, waiting in a fast-food checkout line.

When it comes time to cook the food, take as many shortcuts as you can. Buy pre-cut veggies. At bedtime, move the next night's meat from the freezer to the refrigerator so it's defrosted by dinnertime. Ask your kids and/or spouse to help out in the kitchen. Use a crock pot. Small shortcuts can save a lot of time.

Phase 2: Anchor's away

You've got your PFD, your car stash, your office stash, meals planned for the week and grocery shopping done. Soon, you'll even have your gym bag packed and waiting by the front door (see Chapter 8). Now it's time to launch your new voyage.

Eating do's and don'ts

Do

Measure foods, just at first, until you can eyeball appropriate portions. And get to know your dishes — how many cups do your bowls and glasses hold? Certain foods can be especially deceiving; juice, cereal, nuts, meat, cheese and desserts are some that I recommend measuring a few times. For example, ¼ cup of nuts is about 200 calories. Have you ever taken a ¼ measuring cup and filled it with cashews? There are about 10 cashews in a ¼ cup. So, 20 cashews is 400 calories. That's a lot of calories for a small amount of food. How about cereal? Have you ever used a measuring cup to pour your cereal? The 110 calories in a cup of Cheerios looks awfully small in a big bowl. And when you run out of cereal and you add more for the leftover milk, do you know how much you're adding? Then when you need more milk for that extra cereal, do you know how much you add?

Measuring will help you make educated guesses in the future. A measuring cup is all you need. You may want to also keep a small scale on hand for meats and cheeses, Soon, you won't need to measure or weigh. You'll know how much you're eating just by looking. You're that good. (Although it won't hurt to do a reality check with your measuring cup every once in a while.)

Do

Fix your plate, then put food away. It'll be too much trouble to pick at it then. Family-style eating is great occasionally, but not for every day. It's too easy to go back for seconds.

Do

Create a dining experience. Isn't that one of the reasons you love to go out to eat — for the experience? Your table and your plates are a blank palate just waiting for your personal touch.

When you fix a plate, look at it to see if there's anything you can do to make it more appealing. Can you arrange your vegetables in a pretty pattern? Try cutting fruit in sticks instead of chunks. What about your kitchen? Is it a warm and inviting place to be? Or is it cluttered with junk mail and paperwork? Get all of that mess off of the table and your countertops. Think of the kitchens of friends where you really enjoy spending time. What do they look like? What do they feel like? That's how you want your kitchen to look and feel. Put bright artwork or photos on the walls. Add some plants. Make your kitchen come alive. Your kitchen should be a place where people want to linger over a hot cup of tea or a glass of wine. Consciously turn mealtime into one of the best parts of the day. Take the opportunity to reconnect with loved ones or to be alone with your thoughts. Candles, flowers and pretty place settings can turn a meal into something special, and it doesn't take any extra time. You'll be surprised at your creativity and how much more enjoyable mealtime will be.

Do

Use a plate, not a platter. Use a smaller plate, and you will eat smaller amounts. You'll just think you're eating more.

Do

Stop eating two hours before bedtime. If you're not hungry for breakfast, you're probably eating too much the night before. An article published in a 2007 *International Journal of Obesity* concludes that Night Eating Syndrome (where most food is consumed in the evening and at night) and nocturnal snacking are associated with obesity, binge eating and psychological distress.[13]

Don't

Eat fast food more than one to two times per week. This one is really a no-brainer, isn't it?

Don't

Eat while standing, unless you're a dog or a cat. Sit while you eat. This is a hard one to follow, but you'll be happy you did. Sit. Eat. Enjoy.

Don't

Leave the TV on while you eat. A study published in Bariatric Nursing and Surgical Patient Care in 2007 concluded that viewing television while eating impairs the ability to accurately estimate the total amount of food consumed.[14] Television distracts us, and we may eat more while watching. You can probably live without TV for the time it takes you to eat a meal. If you're used to "noise" while you eat, put on some background music.

Don't

Overdo it. If you haven't prepared your own plate, or if you've helped yourself to seconds, stop halfway through your meal. You've come to the fork in the road, so to speak, so put down your fork and think for a second or two. You have a decision to make. Do you want to clean your plate, or just have a few more bites? Assess the situation and make a conscious decision instead of eating everything in front of you just because it's there. Slow down, stop shoveling, and think about your priorities.

Phase 3: Smooth sailing

Your lifelong journey is under way. You're in the most important phase of the Life Preserver Diet: Smooth Sailing. The Smooth Sailing phase is about following through, remembering your promise to yourself and not giving up. Each day that you spend sailing, the more natural your new lifestyle will feel. You'll get your sea legs! When things get tough, remind yourself that you can do this. When you have a bad day and you've gotten off track, don't give up. (We'll talk more about this in Chapter 9.) All of your planning and preparation will start to pay off. You're in charge now. You're not at the mercy of fast food anymore.

Sometimes you'll want to go back to old habits because it's comfortable. But hey, expand your comfort zone. Your old way of doing things is the old way. It's not part of your reality anymore. The old way got you to a place where you don't want to be. If you continue to do things the old way, there will be no room for the new. Change is hard because we fear the unknown. But, the unknown is exactly what you need right now.

Gone are the days where you binge for months on end. That is the past. It's been too long since you've known what it is like to eat healthy, to feel healthy (and maybe just a little sore from exercise — a good kind of sore), and to wake up in the morning believing that you will succeed. You're no amateur. This is no three-hour tour. You're headed toward a happier, healthier you. Enjoy the cruise.

Chapter 8

The Secret to Exercise:
A little bit every day

This chapter will focus on the who, what, where, when, why and how of exercise.

Who

The first one is easy. **Who** is you.

Of course you're aware of the importance of exercise. But is that enough to get you moving?

Why

Reasons for you to exercise. Let's do a mental exercise together. You don't mind if I get personal, do you? Let's talk about you right now. We know that physical activity is good in general, but how is it good for you, specifically? Think about your reasons for exercising consistently and making it part of your lifestyle.

Think of things that you're not doing now because your weight is holding you back. Visualize yourself in the best shape of your life. What would be different? What are you missing out on? Now, answer this question: "If I were in better shape I would…"

1. _____

2. _____

3. _____

4. _____

5. _____

What did you list? Wear a bikini on the beach? Go on hikes with your family? Stop missing the bus to work? Look back at your answers often. Or write them on a piece of paper and put it in your wallet. This is your future, just waiting for you. Those are your specific Top Five reasons to exercise.

Now for some general reasons why everybody needs to exercise.

1. Balancing intake with outflow.
Calories are the bottom line in weight management. We all like to eat, and we all have our favorite indulgence foods. Mine is cookie dough. I like cookie dough, and sometimes I just gotta have it. It's one of life's little pleasures I really don't want to give up. When I was a little girl, my grandma made great cookies — chocolate chip were my favorite. Every Saturday, she'd get all the ingredients and equipment out, and I'd hang out close enough to grab a few spoonfuls of cookie dough. A few bites of cookie dough can be about 200 calories. So when you just gotta have it, you gotta work it off.

2. A stronger body.
My friend Merrit the boxer says, "You can take the blows much better if you're in shape." That's true for nonboxers, too. Life

throws us a lot of punches. If we're physically strong we're able to bounce back and not be knocked out every time. According to the Mayo Clinic, exercise increases your muscle strength, improves your balance and helps you avoid falls.[15] It can also help you improve your posture, lessen chronic pain and improve your sense of well-being. And there's strong anecdotal evidence to suggest that it keeps us from getting beat up by bullies, too.[16]

3. Preventing chronic disease.

Exercise can help prevent heart disease, cancer, diabetes and so many other health problems. For example, I've got osteoporosis. I don't want it getting any worse. So, I need to take exercise seriously. According to the American Academy of Orthopaedic Surgeons, regular exercise can help reduce the loss of bone mass in older individuals.[17] Improved muscle tone also helps support the skeleton.

What are we doing wrong?

We all make mistakes when it comes to exercising. These are some mistakes to be aware of so you can catch yourself before you make them.

Five things you should not say about exercise:

1. "*Oy*, I'm *schvitzing.*" We tend to think of sweating as a bad thing and say things like, "I'm sweating like a pig." But if we really want to get a good workout in, we've got to work up a sweat. Think of all the toxins you're eliminating and all the endorphins you're releasing when you get a good sweat going. So go ahead, *schvitz!*

2. "I'm just getting old." Let's not confuse getting older with getting out of shape. Have you seen Christie Brinkley lately? Getting older means it gets harder to stay in shape. Age is not on our side. Metabolism slows, schedules get busier, we have more ailments — but that shouldn't be a free pass to slack off. It means we have to work that much harder. Nobody said it was easy.

3. "I'll look stupid doing that." You've got to be willing to look stupid for a while. If you've never done belly dancing before and you decide to take a class, be prepared to look stupid at Lesson 1. If you've never lifted weights and you start to weight train in the gym, you will look out of place until you get the hang of it. If you have never put on roller blades and you go skating in the park, you will look less than graceful at first. It's OK. Most people who catch you looking stupid are going to think to themselves, "Wow, look at that brave person over there, trying something new." And eventually, you'll look less stupid, and you might even find new activities that you really enjoy. But how will you know if you never try?

4. "I'm not athletic." That's a self-fulfilling prophecy. And so is the opposite. If you start telling yourself that you *are* athletic, you will be. With a little practice, you will find the sports goddess within. Get yourself some nice workout clothes, and you're on your way to being an athlete. You are not just working out; you're in training.

5. "I don't like exercise." You shouldn't say this because it is simply not true. You may not like all exercise, but you do like some. Any type of movement or physical activity is exercise. So unless you like to just sit all day, you are not allowed to say this. If you can't find some sort of physical activity that you enjoy —

gardening, walking, playing with your kids or grandkids — then you're not looking hard enough.

Five exercise mistakes:

1. Cheating. Faux Fitness is pretending to work out but never working up a sweat. Sometimes we need to fake it at work, act like we know more than we do until we can look it up. Or on the phone, sounding like we're so happy to hear from someone even though we only picked up because we didn't recognize the number. But one place we must never do this is in the gym. Promise yourself right now that you will not fake it when working out. If we cheat during exercise, we will see very little, if any, results. Instead, be present in the moment and focus on improving your fitness level each time you work out.

2. Thinking of it as a chore. Taking out the garbage is a chore. Paying bills is a chore. But getting fit is a treat. Exercise time is time you take out of your day for your mind, body, spirit. Feel your muscles; be alone with your thoughts; escape the rat race; make yourself healthier; look better; feel stronger; and get ready to take on the world.

3. Believing your own excuses. Don't let yourself off the hook so easily. Do you think you were born yesterday? You do too have time to go, right now. And yes, you'll go tomorrow, but you're going to go today, too. Right?

4. Overlooking little opportunities. Every bit of exercise counts. Taking the stairs instead of the elevator counts. I started doing this because I was claustrophobic and was really afraid to get into elevators. I would go to great lengths to avoid them. People would see me taking the stairs and say, "That's so healthy for you to do that," and I'd smile and agree. But really, it was just because I was terrified of getting in elevators. But then I started realizing how almost everybody I ever walked up stairs with was out of breath after just a few steps. I wasn't. My fear was really working to my advantage. Then I started doing it for exercise. Sometimes, I walk up and down the two flights of stairs in my house for 45 minutes. Or I go to the building next to my office and walk up and down 18 flights, three times. It's a great workout. The stairwell is never crowded, and I only have to do three sets. Talk about *shvitzing*! *Oy!*

Little opportunities for exercise:
- Park in the back of the lot and walk in.
- Get off the bus one stop early.
- Every time you reach the top of your stairs at home, do 10 jumping jacks.
- At the office, don't pick up the phone to talk to co-workers — walk over to their desk.
- Wear ankle weights while you clean the house.

5. Insisting on an all-or-nothing mentality: I used to look at people lifting 3-, 4- and 5-pound weights at the gym and think, "Look at those sissy weights, why even bother? That's not exercising." I told my friend Hayley, a personal trainer, what I thought of those little weights. "Don't knock it till you've tried it," she said. So, I tried it. I started doing sets with those little sissy weights. And I liked them. They helped me keep good form; they were easy on my joints; and they worked! I started noticing results. I bought a whole bunch of sissy weights and put them all over the place. I keep some at my desk at home and at work. Now, I love my sissy weights. I even decorate them for different holidays; little hearts for Valentines Day, fake spiders at Halloween. I take the 3-pounders on trips with me. I've got all different colors. Don't underestimate the power of sissy weights.

How to overcome exercise obstacles

Every day is an obstacle course. We have to jump through a lot of hoops and maneuver around difficult turns to get where we want to go. We can't eliminate all barriers, but we can figure out ways to get around some of them. Here are some tips for overcoming obstacles to fitness.

Obstacle 1: You don't walk enough

Solution: Wear shoes you can actually walk in. Find nice-looking, comfortable shoes and wear them. Because I have a secret to tell you. You don't look as good as you think you do in your heels, unless you're standing still posing for a picture or something. I learned this in Tampa, Fla., 2004. I was traveling through the Tampa airport coming home from a business trip. It's a pretty big airport. I was wearing slingback heels with my tailored black pants and button-down shirt. I thought I looked great, and my legs looked lean and strong, which is pretty much the point of wearing heels. But then I caught a glimpse of myself in a reflection of a store window. I was moving slowly, walking with difficulty, and it wasn't graceful. My feet hurt. There was a long line to get through security. An attractive woman caught my eye in the line next to me. She looked sharp and was nicely dressed. What struck me was that she was walking with such ease and getting through security so smoothly. She took off her shoes and put them in the little bin that goes through the screener. They were Dansko clogs. I got through security without beeping, gathered my bags and put my shoes back on ... but I wished I didn't have to. As I was heading toward Gate 2 grimacing in pain, cursing my slingbacks, I saw Ms. Dansko whizzing by me with her rolling bag, weaving in and out and around people with ease. I was struggling to take each step. I couldn't wait to sit down. I was miserable, and I looked it, too. She was long gone, happily passing all of the gates. I should've snatched her shoes out of the security bin when I had the chance. It was on my way home from that business trip in 2004 that I decided to start wearing comfortable shoes more often and save my heels for special occasions.

Obstacle 2: You have young children at home.

Solution: Get active with your kids. This is a winner for you and your children. Kids imitate our behavior. We can't expect them to be physically active if we're not. Take little ones to the park, or push them in a stroller. Ride bikes with older children, go on hikes or for a swim. It's fun and gives you quality time together. Show them that you value exercise and that being fit is a priority.

Obstacle 3: You can't keep up a regular routine.

Solution: Hire a personal trainer if it helps. Even if you only see a trainer once a month to get ideas and to check in, it can be a great investment. Trainers keep you focused and give you someone to be accountable to.

Obstacle 4: You have trouble staying motivated.

Solution: Consider taking fitness vacations or signing up for a charity walk/run. If you make long-term plans for a specific event, it can help keep you on an exercise schedule and give you something to work toward.

Obstacle 5: Your social life revolves around eating and drinking.

Solution: When you plan to meet friends, get creative. Nothing is wrong with going out to eat with friends, of course. But if you have a lot of friends, that means you're going out to eat a lot. How about meeting a friend for a walk, or going out dancing, or taking an exercise class together? At the very least, meet for a cup of tea instead of ice cream.

Obstacle 6: You don't have the energy to exercise.

Solution: Stop eating junk food; eat to fuel exercise. Once you start working out, you will experience an energy boost. And you will naturally eat healthier because you will crave healthier food. Exercise and energy go hand in hand.

Overcoming the obstacles to fitness is a constant challenge. It's a dynamic process that never ends. But the more practice you get at overcoming these barriers, the easier it becomes.

Where

Where should you exercise? Anywhere and everywhere.

The gym. Just get there, and the rest will take care of itself. You can even multitask while you're there. Listen to music, audio books, or learn Spanish while on the machines ... *Que buena*!

At home. Use workout DVDs and YouTube workouts; add *The Life Preserver Workout* to your home DVD collection. And get a few others, too. You should have a variety so you don't get bored. Between DVD workouts, climb your stairs, mow your lawn, rake leaves, and lift those sissy weights.

Outside. Some days we never make it outside. Be conscious of adding outside activity into your workout repertoire. Walk around the block or go on a jog, a hike, a bike ride.

When can you exercise? Whenever

Working out often ends up on the bottom of our to-do list. It needs to become a priority at the top of our list. Instead of making it the first thing to cut out of a busy day, let it be one of the last. Here are some tips on when to fit it in.

- **During bad TV shows.** Ready to make room for exercise in your life? Then something else has got to go. How will you create a place for exercise? TV is good place to start. Try sticking to only watching your favorite shows. When the boring show comes on, get up and do something. Surfing the Net can get excessive too. If you limit your media time, you'll be able to exchange some media for exercise. Or you can plug in your iPod and take it with you. It's just a matter of changing habits.

- **Right now.** The best time of day to exercise is whenever you can fit it in. I prefer to do it first thing in the morning when I'm too tired to fight it. I put on my workout clothes as soon as I get up, and then I am obligated. But that doesn't always work. So sometimes I have to be flexible and go to plan B (lunch time) or C (after dinner).

- **Tonight.** If your day is almost over and you still haven't worked out, you can do what I call "The Only 20 Workout." Do only 20 minutes of one of the following, or anything you can think of. The best thing about it? It takes only 20 minutes.
  - Jump rope (have you tried it lately?).

- Walk in the neighborhood or on a treadmill.
- Pop in a 20-minute workout DVD.
- Do an upper-body workout with your sissy weights.
- Turn on some music and dance in your living room.
- Walk up and down your stairs.
- Play a round of Wii Fit.

Only 20, and you're done.

Congratulations — you are on your way to becoming an avid exerciser. You will feel and look better than ever. Start with just 20 minutes, and work toward more. The scientists tell us that 60-90 minutes of exercise on most days is what's needed.[18] This science is no joke. We're so off-balance when it comes to living healthy lifestyles. Our sedentary ways have tipped the scales so much that it will take a lot to get where we need to be. But once you start exercising consistently, you will become hooked, and eventually you will meet those guidelines or get close to them.

Now that you know the who, what, where, when, how and why of exercise, you are ready to get started. Remember you chose five things you'd do if you were in better shape. Get ready to do them, because soon you will be in the best shape of your life. Your future is waiting.

The I-mat
Keeping track of your exercise time

As you know from Chapter 5, the PFD keeps track of your food intake and counts any amount of time working out as your exercise. This worksheet will help you build exercise into your routine. Follow this workout for 12 weeks, and before you know it, you'll have formed a good habit.

Don't worry — we don't want to start with that 60- to 90-minute goal. We want to gradually work our way up to 40 minutes day, and we'll consider that a good plateau to stay at for a while. It's all about being your personal best. Keeping track will keep you honest, and you'll be more likely to see results. Remember, it won't be easy. It is doable, though. You are an athlete in training. You can do it. And you may not believe it now, but soon you'll start looking forward to your exercise time.

The I-mat concept. You DO matter. When it comes to exercise, where are you "at"?

Start with 20 minutes of exercise. Then every week, add a little more. Use this form to keep track. When you get to 40 minutes, you're doing great. Sixty minutes (including little exercise opportunities throughout your day) is an excellent long-term goal.

Each day as you carve out your time for exercise, remind yourself: "I-matter." When you've finished your workout, fill in another line below and tell yourself, "I-mat 20 minutes," or "I-mat 22 minutes." You're on your way!

I-mat: Getting up to speed

Week 1: I-mat 20 minutes.

Today I did: (stairs) _____

Today I did: _____

Today I did: _____

Today I did: _____

Today I did: _____

Today I did: _____

Today I did: _____

Week 2: I-mat 22 minutes.

Today I did: _____

Today I did: _____

Today I did: _____

Today I did: _____

Today I did: _____

Today I did: _____

Today I did: _____

I-mat: Getting up to speed (page 2)

Week 3: I-mat 24 minutes.

Today I did: _____

Today I did: _____

Today I did: _____

Today I did: _____

Today I did: _____

Today I did: _____

Today I did: _____

Week 4: I-mat 26 minutes.

Today I did: _____

Today I did: _____

Today I did: _____

Today I did: _____

Today I did: _____

Today I did: _____

Today I did: _____

I-mat: Getting up to speed (page 3)

Week 5: I-mat 28 minutes.

Today I did: _____

Today I did: _____

Today I did: _____

Today I did: _____

Today I did: _____

Today I did: _____

Today I did: _____

Week 6: I-mat 30 minutes!

Today I did: _____

Today I did: _____

Today I did: _____

Today I did: _____

Today I did: _____

Today I did: _____

Today I did: _____

I-mat: Getting up to speed (page 4)

Week 7: I-mat 32 minutes.

Today I did: _____

Today I did: _____

Today I did: _____

Today I did: _____

Today I did: _____

Today I did: _____

Today I did: _____

Week 8: I-mat 34 minutes.

Today I did: _____

Today I did: _____

Today I did: _____

Today I did: _____

Today I did: _____

Today I did: _____

Today I did: _____

I-mat: Getting up to speed (page 5)

Week 9: I-mat 36 minutes.

Today I did: _____

Today I did: _____

Today I did: _____

Today I did: _____

Today I did: _____

Today I did: _____

Today I did: _____

Week 10: I-mat 38 minutes.

Today I did: _____

Today I did: _____

Today I did: _____

Today I did: _____

Today I did: _____

Today I did: _____

Today I did: _____

I-mat: Getting up to speed (page 6)

Week 11: I-mat 40 minutes!

Today I did: _____

Today I did: _____

Today I did: _____

Today I did: _____

Today I did: _____

Today I did: _____

Today I did: _____

Week 12: I-mat 40 minutes (& holding)

Today I did: _____

Today I did: _____

Today I did: _____

Today I did: _____

Today I did: _____

Today I did: _____

Today I did: _____

Worksheet: Keep your eye on the prize

Worthy goals are difficult, specific and achievable. They start with baby steps and end with a motivating challenge: a Fourth of July fun-run, for instance, or looking your best for an upcoming college reunion.

Set a few specific, achievable goals for yourself. What are you going to do with all this fitness? Learn to tango? Climb to the top of the Eiffel Tower? Race your nephew at the park, and win?

List them here:

1. _____

2. _____

3. _____

Chapter 9

Man Overboard!
When your direction has taken a turn for the worse

When someone screams, "MAN OVERBOARD!" it's not taken lightly. I admit, I've never actually heard anyone scream that, but if I did, I imagine that drastic measures would be taken to get the person out of the dangerous waters and back on board to safety.

We all fall off of our plan at some point. That's to be expected — the challenges of our everyday lives send us over the edge sometimes. We feel like we're doing everything we can just to survive … like we're barely hanging on. But when we do find ourselves overboard, we may have to take some drastic measures to get out of the predicament — or we may spend weeks or months adrift until we can get back on board.

OK, here my "overboard" metaphor may start to fall apart … but when it comes to changing your eating and exercise habits, there are degrees of overboardness. Going overboard on a cruise may be an all-or-nothing thing, but with eating and exercising, you might just have a bad day — or you might have a bad month. Either way, I've got some tips to help you get back on course.

Green alert: You've plateaued

Maybe you've had some success so far, but all of a sudden, your scale won't budge and your clothes don't look any looser. You're starting to feel discouraged. What can you do?

Whine. It's good to be grateful for what you've got, but occasionally, don't we all just need a good whining session? I know I do. For me, that's when my "Trouble with Today" list comes in handy. I write down all the things that are bugging me for that day — even things like, "My favorite jeans still don't fit!" Just getting it off my chest makes me feel better. It's like a good cry.

Get out a tape measure. The scale is important; it keeps us honest. We all want to see those numbers go down. But it's not the only way to measure weight-loss success. Sometimes we lose inches before weight, especially if we're exercising regularly. The way your clothes fit, your energy level and how you feel about yourself are equally important. Try not to dwell on the scale. If you keep on track, the scale will eventually cooperate.

Laugh. Remember Morgan Freeman's character in the movie, "*The Bucket List?*" He said that before he died, he wanted to laugh so hard that he cried. Shouldn't we all do that more? Of course we should; laughing is one life's great joys. It's fun, it reduces stress, brings people together and helps us maintain a healthy weight. Researchers from Vanderbilt University found that if you laugh for 10 minutes a day, you can burn 50 calories — which adds up to 5 pounds in a year.[19] It's time to start hanging out with your funny friends. If you don't have any, find yourself some.

Have a pity party. But don't keep the decorations up too long. Hey, no one said it was going to be easy. You've worked hard, and you deserve results! But take a closer look. You're getting results: You've got more energy, don't you? You're proud of what you've accomplished so far, aren't you? Just keep at it, and you'll reach all your goals.

Keep it all in perspective. Keep in mind that you can eat anything you want; it's just a matter of how much, how often. No room on your on your PFD for a little treat? Don't worry; there'll be three more "extra" shares tomorrow.

Reassess. Take a day to really watch what you eat, and how you account for it on your PFD. Maybe you're eating more than you think.

- If you notice that you're "sampling" while you cook, for instance, have some crudités of raw veggies out and ready to munch, or whip up a Don't Blow It Now Shake (see recipe in Chapter 10).

- If you can't stop munching after dinner, chew mint flavored gum. Or brush your teeth. Nothing tastes good after that.

- If you're at work and you crave sugar in the afternoons, it's time to replenish your office stash.

- If you haven't been drinking enough water, start! Over the past 37 years, the number of calories adults get through beverages has almost doubled, according to a study by Barry M. Popkin, professor of nutrition at the Carolina Population Center.[20] Water, on the other hand, is calorie-free.

Blue alert: You've lost the wind in your sails

Maybe you had some success but then you let your guard down.
Or maybe you've just lost your inspiration. Either way, you're
feeling uninspired. Don't give up now! Here are a few tips to get
back on track:

- Carry your bathing suit in your purse.

- Buy some Spanx (body shapers). It'll help smooth out your rear
  view.

- Call, text or e-mail someone who can talk some sense into you
  when you find yourself slipping.

- Recognize when you're falling back into old habits. Don't let
  them win.

- Do it for the children. They're watching your every move — be
  a good role model.

- Live in the moment and enjoy the process. You'll appreciate all
  that you do have and not worry so much about what you don't
  have yet.

- If you eat big lunches with clients or at meetings, have a teeny
  tiny dinner (about 300 calories, or three shares). That will help
  balance out your calories for the day.

- If you tend to look for food when you're not hungry, put a note
  on the inside of the fridge that says, "What are you looking
  for?" "Are you sure it's in here?"

Yellow alert: You've lost your will to move

You're sticking to your PFD; you're eating right, but what happened to the exercise? Somehow, you stopped making time to exercise a little, every day. Or maybe you never got started, and now it's caught up to you because you've stopped losing weight. That's to be expected: For long-term weight loss and long-term healthy living, a good diet and regular exercise must go hand in hand (so true!). In the weight loss game, you've got to always trick your body into thinking it's NOT starving. If you cut your food intake, it will adjust to a lower metabolic rate to make up for the fewer calories. When you exercise, you rev up your metabolic rate, and your body can't help but burn calories. Plus, once you get used to getting a little sweaty, exercise feels GOOD. Your body craves movement, so give it what it wants.

- **If you're not going, ask yourself why.** Do you belong to a gym that's convenient for you? Is it close to home? Are the hours working for you? If not, join another one.

- **Get a jump start.** Sign up for that charity walk you've wanted to do, a 5k, gym membership, spin class, belly-dancing or personal trainer, anything that gets you moving. In fact, maybe you should put this book down right now and sign up for something immediately. Go ahead, I'll wait right here.

- **Let's talk about your bag.** When you are prepared for the gym, you will be more likely to go on a regular basis. What goes in the gym bag? I can tell you because I am an organized gym bag packer. But I wasn't always. In the past, when I would shower at the gym after a workout, it was a free-for-all. I'd inevitably forget to pack something crucial: panties, a towel, a comb. It never failed. But there was a woman who was in the locker room every day at the same time as me. She would unpack exactly what she needed, and she looked completely pulled together when she left. I asked her what her secret was. Turns out she is a professional organizer (what are the chances?) and she generously offered me her tips. Now, I'm passing them on to you!

Some ideas for an organized gym bag (adapted from professional organizer Suellen Germani). A rolling bag is easiest to transport from car to gym.

Lock for gym locker
Shorts/tights/sweat pants
T-shirt
Sports bra
Shoes and socks
Towel to dry sweat off equipment if not provided
         by the gym.
Any workout notes not stored at the gym
Fingerless gloves if lifting weights
Water bottle
MP3 player
Shampoo and conditioner
Soap
Razor
Shaving cream
Moisturizer/lotion
Deodorant
Hair gel/spray
Hair brush/comb
Blow dryer, if not provided by the gym
Make up and other hair accessories

Change of clothing
Street shoes and socks, pantyhose
Underwear
Bra
A mini makeup bag

- **Review your workout routine.** Are you working hard enough? Have you mixed up your workout routines lately? Are you checking your heart rate? We tend to get a little too comfortable in our exercise routine and wonder why we aren't getting the results we want. Challenge yourself by trying something new.

- **Look for opportunities everywhere.** When we work on computers all day, we can easily forget to get up and move around. I was guilty of this. So, I decided to take my stapler off of my desk and put it in the office copy room. Now, every time I have to staple something, I take about 50 steps, round trip. If I staple eight times a day, I've walked an extra 400 steps. That equals 2,000 steps or 1 mile per week. Moving my stapler allowed me to walk an extra mile each week. I'll take it. Every little bit counts.

- **Plan for the holidays.** When Halloween approaches, get ready. You're going to eat more calories, probably for a couple of months. There really is no way around it. A study published in *The New England Journal of Medicine* said that Americans gain a small amount of weight every holiday season.[21] Because it's a small amount, one to two pounds, we tend to let it slide. So the weight keeps creeping on, year after year. What are we to do? Avoid all holiday parties and family gatherings from November to January? Not a good idea. That may cause you to end up depressed at home drowning your sorrows with spiked eggnog and rum balls. Instead, say yes to holiday cheer and start burning more calories ahead of time. Don't wait until New Year's Day. Start increasing the frequency, intensity and duration of your exercise on Halloween. Add 15 or 20 minutes each time you go to the gym, take an additional class or buy a new fitness DVD (and use it). Do something to take it up a notch before the holidays begin. Keep it up through the season. Come Jan. 1, you'll be way ahead of the game.

Orange alert: You're overwhelmed!

Life is crazy enough, and who has time for this life preserver stuff, anyway? Well, you do. But perhaps you've temporarily forgotten how much you deserve good food and a fit body, amid all the kids' needs and driving everywhere and busy, busy days. Don't fret. Follow these tips to refocus and get back with the program for a happier, healthier you:

- **Give yourself a "me day."** When is the last time you took a day off just for you? Well, now there's one day on your calendar with your name on it. Do whatever you want with that time. Clean out your closet, empty your inbox, go through your bills, make doctor's appointments, see a movie, get your nails done or just have a lazy day. Keep one day out of the month open for an appointment with yourself so you can stay on top of your life. But try to make it to your own appointment. You don't want to stand yourself up. Once you get in this habit, you're going to love it. I promise.

- **Take a nap.** You know you need one.

- **If you cannot find any time to cook, have your spouse do**

it for you. Or give the kids a chore, if they're old enough: Each kid gets to make dinner one night a week. (If you're still cooking too much, have more kids!)

- **Take a no-phone day.** Just turn it off. No one will know. If anyone asks where you were, say you left your phone in your car. You can call them back later, once you've gotten back on track with your good-food-happy-body lifestyle.

- **Hire a cleaning service,** even if you can only afford one day every once in a while. Anyone can clean your house for you, but only you can exercise for you.

- **Don't ever give in.** Nothing and no one can stop you.

Red alert! You've fallen, and you can't get up

You're not sure how or when it happened, but one day, you just stopped keeping track with your PFD. And then, one day you forgot to go to the gym, and you never went again. I'm here to tell you … whether it's been two weeks, two months or two years, it's not too late. You can get back on course, and you can do it right now.

- **Change your environment.** I highly recommend girls' trips. Two of my best friends and I have been going on an annual getaway for as long as I can remember. We call them our ego-maintenance trips. It's something we absolutely make time for each year. No excuses. It's three days of laughing, relaxing and just letting our hair down, usually at a beach. I find my sense of humor again, and I breathe a little deeper. After a day or two I start remembering how funny, charming, and intelligent I am.

By the end of the trip, I feel like a million bucks. I'm ready to return to my real life and face any challenge head-on. It might be time for you to take an emergency ego-maintenance getaway. "Marcia, are you crazy?" you ask. "I barely have time to do my laundry; how do you think I'm going to find time to plan a trip?" Surely you have time to call a friend, pick a date, get it on the calendar and work out the details later. You don't even have to go far or spend lots of money. Stay overnight at a local hotel with your honey, or swap homes for a weekend with a friend. We're never gonna survive unless we get a little crazy. If that's not reason enough, consider this: A vacation may keep you from having a heart attack. According to a multiyear study by Brooks B. Gump, an associate professor of psychology at State University of New York, people who skipped taking a vacation for five straight years were 30 percent more likely to have a heart attack than those who took one every year.[22]

- **If cooking is getting you down,** go through your recipe files/books and replace old recipes that you never use with new, interesting recipes that you want to try.

- **If you find it hard to control portions at restaurants,** sabotage your food. That's right, go for it. When you know you've had enough, put a sugar packet on your fries or salt on your cheesecake. Do whatever it takes to make your food less appetizing. Just for fun, do it nonchalantly and see whether anyone comments.

- **If you travel often,** stock your hotel room with food upon your arrival so that you only eat out once a day.

Feeling better?

Now you're back on board. You're going to be fine.

Celebrate! Here's to you — the one who hit some choppy waters or even fell overboard. You took control and got yourself out of harm's way. It's not the first time you struggled, and it won't be the last. But from this day forward you will do whatever it takes to save yourself. You're ready to take the helm, turn this vessel around and start heading in the right direction. The future is looking bright.

Glad to have you back.

Chapter 10

Navigating the Kitchen
Recipes to get you started

Fact is, it's a lot easier to lose weight when you make your meals yourself. When you cook, you're in control. You know exactly how much fat you're putting in there; you know exactly how much beef or rice you've made. The minor inconvenience of preparing the food (and trust us, most take-out orders take longer than the recipes described here) is far offset by the convenience of better managing your meals. Besides, it's a well-known rule that if you also cook for someone else while you're at it, that someone else has to do the dishes. So go ahead, make a mess!

The recipes included here are not meant to be repeated day in and day out, like magic potions that will automatically make you lose weight. They are meant as suggestions to get your creative juices flowing, and as examples to show you how to allocate PFD shares. Give them a whirl, and then modify them to suit your tastes, or try something entirely new.

Breakfast

Scrambled Eggs with Shiitake Mushrooms and Herbs

Mushrooms are a natural partner for eggs, and shiitakes are an especially good match because their texture is soft and their flavor is subtle. Plus, they add extra bulk to your eggs to give you more food on your plate. Serve over whole wheat toast or a bed of steamed spinach.

2 servings   Hands on: 15 minutes   Total time: 15 minutes

    8 ounces fresh shiitake mushrooms
    1 teaspoon olive oil
    Salt and pepper
    4 eggs (or 2 eggs plus 2 egg whites)
    Pinch nutmeg (freshly grated is best)
    1 tablespoon minced fresh parsley
    1 tablespoon minced fresh chives

Remove the stems from the mushrooms and discard (or save
for a soup stock). Slice the caps into 1/2-inch wide strips. Heat
the oil in a sauté pan over medium-high heat and add the
mushrooms. Sprinkle with salt and pepper. Cook for 3-4 minutes
without stirring. Turn and cook an additional 2-3 minutes,
until mushrooms are tender. Transfer to a bowl and set aside.
In a separate bowl, lightly whisk the eggs with the nutmeg and
a pinch each of salt and pepper. Return the sauté pan used to
cook the mushroom to medium-low heat. Add the eggs. Add the
mushrooms and herbs; stir gently with a nonstick spatula until
eggs are thick and creamy, 3-5 minutes.

Shares per serving
    meat & beans: 1
    veggies: 1

Apple Fennel Breakfast Salad

Fennel is a big bulb, kinda celery-like, with a slight licorice flavor.
Don't be scared! It's refreshing and not overpowering, and it pairs
especially well with orange or apple. Feel free to vary the fruits
and nuts in this recipe to your own taste.

4 servings   Hands on: 10 minutes   Total time: 10 minutes

 2 apples, quartered, cored and chopped into slices
 1 bulb fennel, trimmed, quartered, hard white core removed,
    and thinly sliced crosswise (into thin crescent shapes)
 2 tablespoons golden raisins
 2 tablespoons chopped walnuts
 1 cup nonfat plain or vanilla yogurt
 1 tablespoon honey

In a large bowl, combine all ingredients.

Shares per serving
   veggies: 1
   fruit: 1

Lunch

Santa Fe Salad

The great thing about this salad is that it uses no dressing — just store-bought salsa, which is almost always fat free (and so much lower in calories, and higher in nutrients, than typical salad dressings). Mix and match ingredients depending on what you have available.

In my opinion, a salad spinner is an essential piece of kitchen equipment. Mine gets used at least once a day to quickly rinse and dry leafy vegetables of all kinds.

1 serving   Hands on: 20 minutes (or less)
Total time: 30 minutes

4 cups mixed lettuce and/or spinach leaves, rinsed and
  spun dry
1/4 cup canned black or pinto beans, rinsed and drained
1 ounce cooked, sliced chicken breast
  (see *How to Cook a Chicken Breast*)
1 Roma tomato, chopped
A few thin slices red onion
1 carrot, chopped
4 mushrooms, sliced
1 tablespoon chopped fresh herbs — oregano, marjoram,
  basil, cilantro and/or thyme
1/4 teaspoon cumin seeds
1/4 cup salsa

Place the salad greens in a bowl (or plastic container with a lid).
Top with remaining ingredients. Toss before serving.

Shares per serving
  meat & beans: 1
  veggies: 3

How to cook a chicken breast

This speedy, no-thrills method comes in handy for salads,
sandwiches, pasta dishes and soups.

1 whole chicken breast (two halves), skinless and boneless

Place the chicken breast in a saucepan and cover with water.
Cover and bring to a boil over high heat. Reduce the heat slightly
to prevent boiling over. Cook 15-20 minutes, until the chicken
is cooked through (it will appear solid white in the center when
pierced with a knife). Remove from heat; remove the chicken

from the water and place on a plate or cutting board to cool. When the chicken is cool enough to handle, use a sharp knife to cut it into slices. If desired, use your kitchen scale to divide the slices into 2-ounce groups; pack in individual containers or resealable baggies.

If you cook a lot of chicken at once, you can use the cooking water to make a quick soup. After removing the chicken, add some diced carrot, diced celery and diced onion to the broth. Bring to a simmer and cook until the vegetables are tender, about 10 minutes. Season to taste with salt and pepper; dice some of the cooked chicken and add it to the pot. *Voila*, chicken soup!

Super Shreddy Veggie Sandwich

When you're in a shreddin' mood, go ahead and shred a bunch of stuff and store it in the fridge. You can use it on sandwiches and salads for several days.

1 serving   Hands on: 5 minutes   Total time: 5 minutes

    1 small whole wheat pita pocket or 1/2 large whole wheat
        pita pocket
    1 cup shredded fresh raw vegetables, any combination of the
        following: beet (scrubbed, roots and stem trimmed), carrot,
        jicama (peeled first), broccoli stem, kohlrabi, cabbage or
        romaine lettuce
    1 ounce shredded cheese
    2-3 slices tomato (optional)
    1 slice onion (optional)
    bean sprouts or alfalfa sprouts (optional)
    1 tablespoon salad dressing, any kind

Stuff the pita pocket with the shredded vegetables and cheese. Top with tomato, onion and sprouts, if desired. Drizzle with salad dressing.

Shares per serving
dairy: 1
whole grains: 1
veggies: 2

Tomato Soup and Popcorn

This is one of the best — and fastest — lunches of all time. Make your co-workers jealous with your big bowl of popcorn! And no, you don't have to share.

    1 single-serving bag plain microwave popcorn
    1/4 cup grated Parmesan cheese
    1 tablespoon chopped fresh rosemary
    1 bowl tomato soup (canned, boxed, whatever you've got)
    1 ounce shredded cooked chicken, turkey, beef or ham,
        or 1/4 cup canned rinsed beans

Cook the popcorn according to package directions. When it's done, add the Parmesan and rosemary, then close the bag tightly and shake well to combine. Heat the tomato soup and add the shredded meat or beans. Top with a handful of popcorn, if desired.

Shares per serving
meat & beans: 1
dairy: 1
whole grains: 1
veggies: 2

Snacks

Don't-Blow-It-Now Shake

So easy, so satisfying! Use what you've got handy, and eat this instead of something you'll regret later.

1 serving   Hands on: 5 minutes   Total time: 5 minutes

Choose one of the following:
>   1 cup frozen fruit: strawberries, blueberries, peaches, mangoes, blackberries, etc. (or any combination)
>   1 banana
>   1 cup fresh fruit

Place in a blender. Add a handful of ice cubes. Cover, then blend for 30 seconds.

Add one of the following:
>   1 cup skim milk
>   6 oz. nonfat yogurt
>   1 cup plain soy milk
>   1 cup rice or almond milk

Cover and blend until smooth. For variety, add one (or all) of the following:
>   1/2 teaspoon vanilla extract
>   1/4 teaspoon almond extract
>   1 tablespoon unsweetened cocoa powder
>   1 teaspoon honey

Shares per serving
>   dairy: 1
>   fruit: 1

C.R O. Muffins

Looking for a hardy snack? These muffins have less fat than the store-bought kind plus lots of fill-you-up fiber in the oats and carrots.

12 muffins   Hands on: 35 minutes   Total time: 40 minutes

    1 cup all-purpose flour
    3/4 cup rolled oats
    1 teaspoon baking powder
    3/4 teaspoon baking soda
    1 1/2 teaspoons ground cinnamon
    1/2 teaspoon salt
    2 eggs (or egg whites)
    3/4 cup packed brown sugar
    1/4 cup vegetable oil
    1/2 cup apple sauce
    1 teaspoon vanilla
    2 large carrots, grated or chopped finely in a food processor
    1/2 cup raisins

Preheat the oven to 350 degrees. Line 12 muffin cups with paper cupcake liners. In a large bowl, combine the flour, oats, baking powder, baking soda, cinnamon and salt. In a small bowl, beat the eggs, then stir in the brown sugar, oil, apple sauce and vanilla. Add the wet ingredients to the dry and stir just until combined. Stir in the carrots and raisins. Divide the batter among the muffin cups. Bake 18 to 20 minutes, until the muffins spring back when lightly touched in the center.

Shares per serving
whole grains: 1
extra: 1

Broiled Grapefruit

A fancy (and fun) way to eat your fruit!

1 serving   Hands on: 5 minutes   Total time: 15 minutes

1/2 large grapefruit, cut crosswise
1 teaspoon packed brown sugar
1 maraschino cherry (optional)

Place a rack in your oven 6 inches from the broiler; preheat the broiler. Meanwhile, using a serrated knife, carefully cut the grapefruit sections around the membranes to loosen. Leave the sections in the grapefruit shell.

Place the grapefruit half, cut side up, on an oven-safe baking dish or pan. Sprinkle evenly with the brown sugar. Cook a few inches under the broiler for 3-5 minutes, until top is slightly browned and bubbly (but not burned!). Remove from the oven; place cherry in center.

Shares per serving
fruit: 1

Dinner

Pasta With Peas and Prosciutto

This creamless version of the classic Tuscan combination has less fat but plenty of flavor. Since you're only using a little bit of prosciutto (an Italian cured ham), you'll probably want to opt for a good-quality imported brand.

Makes 4 servings   Hands on: 20 minutes

Hands on: 25 minutes

  12 ounces dried pasta, such as bow-tie or penne
  1 cup fresh or frozen English peas
  1 tablespoon butter
  1 large shallot, peeled and finely chopped
  2 ounces prosciutto, chopped
  1/2 cup defatted chicken or vegetable stock
  1/2 teaspoon nutmeg
  Kosher salt and freshly ground black pepper to taste
  1/2 cup grated Parmesan cheese

Bring a large pot of water to boil. Add pasta and cook until al dente. Add peas and cook until 30 more seconds. Drain in a colander.

Meanwhile, melt butter in a large skillet over medium-high heat. Add shallots and prosciutto until shallots soften, 3-4 minutes. Add chicken stock and boil until liquid is reduced by about half. Add pasta and peas and toss. Season with nutmeg, salt and pepper. Serve with cheese.

Shares per serving
  whole grains: 3 (whole wheat pasta)
  extra: 3 (white pasta)

The Art of Stir-fry

Stir-frying — fast-frying over high heat — is just an easy, versatile way to have a hot meal and use up all those vegetables in your refrigerator. Your ultimate goal is to end up with a big bowl of hot, tender-crisp vegetables, plus a little sauce for flavor and maybe some meat or tofu for protein. If you don't have time to cook brown rice, consider serving your stir-fry over quinoa — it's a whole grain, like brown rice, but it only takes 15 minutes to cook. You can usually find quinoa in the healthy food section of your grocery store.

Since the only no-no when stir-frying is to overcook the veggies, here are a few tips to keep the process running smoothly.

- Never, ever measure anything. It ruins the fun!

- Choose just a few vegetables, so you can enjoy the flavor of each.

- Before you start chopping, put your rice or quinoa on, or start the water boiling for soba noodles. By the time you get everything prepared for the wok, your rice or noodles will be just about ready.

- Make sure all ingredients are ready to go before you start stir-frying.

- If you have a wok, heat it for a minute or two before you add the oil. If you're using a frying pan with nonstick coating, heat the oil with the pan to prevent damage to the coating (follow manufacturer's directions).

- Choose an oil with a high smoke point, like refined peanut, canola or safflower.

- If you're using meat or tofu, cube it and cook it separately, then set it aside while you cook the vegetables. The reason is that you generally want your protein to cook to a nice, golden color —

but you don't want your vegetables to brown.

- Don't overload your wok or frying pan. Stir-fried food must come in direct contact with the sizzling-hot pan. If necessary, cook in batches.

- Start with the longest-cooking vegetables first, like carrots, onions, green beans, bell peppers. If you're uncertain about the order in which to stir-fry vegetables, stir-fry them one at a time, and then toss them all in the pan at the end to reheat.

- Keep the ingredients moving to prevent browning.

- When adding a sauce that needs to thicken, push the other ingredients up the sides of the pan to create an open well in the middle. Add the sauce, stir until it thickens, and then stir the other ingredients into it.

- Serve stir-fry immediately, while it's hot and before vegetables get soft.

A few combos to try:

- Asparagus, red bell peppers, mushrooms, garlic, soy sauce over brown rice

- Yukon gold potatoes, Swiss chard, dried cherries, ginger, plum sauce over quinoa

- Butternut squash, onion, spinach, ginger, soy sauce, and a touch of chili paste over soba noodles

Vegetable and Soba Noodle Bowl

With red peppers, yellow squash and bright green snow pea pods, what could be prettier than this simple sitr fry? And when it's seasoned with fresh ginger and garlic, what could be tastier?

Makes 4 servings   Hands on: 25 minutes
Total time: 25 minutes

> 8 ounces soba noodles
> 2 tablespoons canola oil
> 8 ounces diced chicken or tofu
> 2 large red bell peppers, cut into thin strips
> 8 ounces sliced mushrooms
> 1/4 cup fresh peeled chopped ginger
> 3 large cloves garlic, minced
> 2 medium yellow squash, thinly sliced
> 3 tablespoons low-sodium soy sauce
> 1 cup chicken or vegetable broth
> 2 teaspoons balsamic vinegar
> 2 cups snow peas, trimmed
> 1/3 cup chopped cilantro
> 2 green onions, thinly sliced

Bring a large pot of water to boil. In the meantime, prepare vegetables. When the water comes to a boil, add the soba noodles and cook just to al dente (be careful not to overcook). Drain.

Heat 1 tablespoon of the oil in a large wok over medium high heat. Add the chicken or tofu and stir fry until lightly browned. Remove from pan and set aside. Add the remaining tablespoon of oil to the wok. Saute bell peppers, shiitake mushrooms, ginger and garlic for 3 minutes. Add squash, tamari, broth and vinegar.

Cook 3 minutes. Stir in snow peas, cilantro and green onions, sauté 2-3 minutes until snow peas are bright green. Return the chicken or tofu to the pan, and then add the noodles. Serve warm or at room temperature.

Shares per serving
  meat & beans: 1
  whole grains: 1
  veggies: 2

Spinach-Stuffed Pork Tenderloin

You can "stuff" (roll, really) pork tenderloin with just about anything — chopped apples and pine nuts, for instance, or chopped vegetables, cheeses, other meats. Spinach is another good choice.

3 to 4 servings   Hands on: 15 minutes
Total time: 35 minutes

  1 teaspoon olive oil
  1 clove garlic, minced
  4 cups fresh spinach, rinsed and dried
  1 tablespoon chopped fresh marjoram
  1 tablespoon chopped sun-dried tomatoes
  4 kalamata olives, pitted and chopped
  Salt and freshly ground pepper to taste
  1 pork tenderloin
  1 tablespoon freshly grated Parmesan cheese

Preheat the oven to 400 degrees. In a large skillet, heat the oil over medium-high heat. Add the garlic and cook for 30 seconds. Stir in the spinach and cook until wilted. Add the marjoram, sun-dried tomatoes and olives and season to taste with salt and pepper. Set aside.

Cut the pork tenderloin lengthwise without cutting all the way through; open and flatten the tenderloin. Pound it with a meat mallet to 1/4-inch thickness.

Spread the spinach mixture over the tenderloin and sprinkle with the Parmesan cheese. Roll it lengthwise, like a jelly roll, and tie with kitchen twine. Place on in a shallow roasting pan or baking dish.

Roast for 20-25 minutes until juices run clear (internal temperature should reach 160 degrees). Remove from oven, remove string and slice crosswise into rounds.

Shares per serving
meat & beans: 2
veggies: 1

Endnotes

1. Christine Lagorio. 2005. "Diet Plan Success Tough to Weigh," Associated Press.

2. "FRONTLINE" April 9, 2004 Diet Wars

3. Gallup-Healthways Well-Being Index, Feb. 10, 2011.

4. Powell, de Lemos, Banks, Ayers, Rohatgi, Khera, McGuire, Berry, Albert, Vega, Grundy and Sandeep R. Das. 2010. "Body Size Misperception: A Novel Determinant in the Obesity Epidemic." Arch Intern Med 170(18):1695-1697. doi:10.1001/archinternmed.2010.314.

5. Finkelstein, DiBonaventura, Burgess, Somali and Brent C. Hale. 2010. "The Costs of Obesity in the Workplace," *Journal of Occupational & Environmental Medicine* 52: 971-976. doi: 10.1097/JOM.0b013e3181f274d2.

6. Heiland and Mary Burke. 2007. "Social Dynamics of Obesity." *Academic Journal of Economic Inquiry* 45: 571-591.

7. Byrne, Cooper and C. Fairburn. 2003. "Weight Maintenance and relapse in obesity: a qualitative study." *International Journal of Obesity* 27: 955-962.

8. Kruger, Blanck and Cathleen Gillespie. 2006. "Dietary and physical activity behaviors among adults successful at weight loss maintenance." *International Journal of Behavioral Nutrition and Physical Activity* 3:17 doi:10.1186/1479-5868-3-17

9. The National Lung and Blood Institute. "Obesity Guidelines." Accessed 2011. http://natamcancer.org/handouts/Gov-AHA_PDF_prev_earlydetection/NHLBI_HealthyFoodShopping.pdf

10. Spiegel, Tasali, Penev and E Van Cavter. 2004. "Brief Communication: Sleep Curtailment in Healthy Young Men Is Associated with Decreased Leptin Levels, Elevated Ghrelin levels and Increased Hunger and Appetite." *Annals of Internal Medicine.* 141:1-52.

11. Gary D. Foster. 2006. "Clinical Implications for the Treatment of Obesity." *Obesity Research.* 14:182-185.

12. Mancino and Jean Kinsey. 2008. "Is Dietary Knowledge Enough? Hunger, Stress and Other Roadblocks to Healthy Eating. *USDA Economic Research.* 62: 1-20.

13. Colles, Dixon, and PE O'Brien. 2007. " Night Eating Syndrome and Nocturnal Snacking: association with obesity, binge eating and psychological distress." *International Journal of Obesity.* 31:1722-1730.

14. Moray, Fu, Brill and Monica S. Mayoral. 2007. "Viewing Television While Eating Impairs the Ability to Accurately Estimate Total Amount of Food Consumed." *Bariatric Nursing and Surgical Patient Care.* 2: 71-76.

15. Mayo Foundation for Medical Education and Research. 2008

16. We're kidding. There's no such study!

17. American Academy of Orthopedic Surgeons. 2007. http://orthoinfo.aaos.org/topic.cfm?topic=a00232.

18. United States Department of Agriculture *2010 Dietary Guidelines for Americans.*

19. Buchowski, Majchrzak, Bloomquist, Chen, Byrne and JA Backorowski. 2007. "Energy Expenditure of Genuine Laughter." *International Journal of Obesity.* 31:131-137.

20. Popkin and S. Nielsen. 2001. "Changes in Beverage Intake Between 1977 and 2001." *American Journal of Preventitive Medicine.* 27: 205-210.

21. Yanovski, Zanovski, Sovik, Nguyen, O'Neil and Nancy G. Sevring. 2000. "A Prospective Study of Holiday Weight Gain." *The New England Journal of Medicine.* 342: 861-867.

22. Gump and Karen A Mathews. 2000. "Are Vacations Good for your Health? The 9 year Mortality Experience After the Multiple Risk Factor Intervention Trial." *Psychosomatic Medicine.* 62: 608-612.

About the Authors

Marcia Berlin is a registered dietitian, a professional speaker, a cancer survivor, a working mom, a fitness instructor and a former professional dancer. As the onsite dietitian at DeKalb Medical Center's Wellness Center in Decatur, Ga., she offered diet and nutrition advice to thousands of people. As a popular public speaker and the Atlanta Regional Commission's health and wellness specialist, she gives about 20 speeches a year on health issues. And as a breast cancer survivor and pioneer among cancer gene carriers for preventative surgery (double mastectomy/hysterectomy), she knows firsthand the value of good health and the importance of choosing a healthy lifestyle.

Over the past decade, Berlin has earned a reputation as an engaging and dynamic public speaker. She wins over her audiences with her enthusiasm and illustrates her message with creative demonstrations — often charming audience members into acting as genes, blood cells or sandwich makers. Health administrators and corporate event organizers know to call on Berlin for lively, enlightening presentations.

Consulting author **Deborah Geering** is a professional writer and editor with a special interest in food writing. After 15 years in newspapers as a copy editor, supervisory editor and section editor, she launched a freelance reporting career in 2001. For eight years, she wrote weekly food articles for *The Atlanta Journal-Constitution*'s award-winning food section, often creating and testing the accompanying recipes and styling them for photographs. Currently, she is a contributing editor to

Atlantamagazine.com, where she writes a weekly blog about local food. A veteran vegetarian, Deborah has developed and produced a vegetarian cooking column called The Veggie Life. She has been published in magazines including *People, Cooking Light, Georgia Magazine,* and *Atlanta Magazine,* as well as other outlets including USAToday.com, Fodor's travel books, and several business publications. A daily devotee of her local YMCA, she has collaborated with co-author Marcia Berlin on newspaper articles about nutrition and healthy lifestyles.

12147357R00092

Made in the USA
Lexington, KY
28 November 2011